Disaster Mental Health: Around the World and Across Time

Editors

CRAIG L. KATZ
ANAND PANDYA

PSYCHIATRIC CLINICS OF NORTH AMERICA

www.psych.theclinics.com

September 2013 • Volume 36 • Number 3

ELSEVIER

1600 John F. Kennedy Boulevard • Suite 1800 • Philadelphia, Pennsylvania, 19103-2899

http://www.theclinics.com

PSYCHIATRIC CLINICS OF NORTH AMERICA Volume 36, Number 3
September 2013 ISSN 0193-953X, ISBN-13: 978-0-323-18870-8

Editor: Joanne Husovski
Developmental Editor: Donald Mumford

Psychiatric Clinics of North America (ISSN 0193-953X) is published quarterly by Elsevier Inc., 360 Park Avenue South, New York, NY 10010-1710. Months of issue are March, June, September, and December. Business and Editorial Offices: 1600 John F. Kennedy Blvd., Suite 1800, Philadelphia, PA 19103-2899. Periodicals postage paid at New York, NY and additional mailing offices. Subscription prices are $286.00 per year (US individuals), $524.00 per year (US institutions), $141.00 per year (US students/residents), $347.00 per year (Canadian individuals), $651.00 per year (Canadian Institutions), $431.00 per year (foreign individuals), $651.00 per year (foreign institutions), and $210.00 per year (international & Canadian students/residents). Foreign air speed delivery is included in all *Clinics'* subscription prices. All prices are subject to change without notice. **POSTMASTER:** Send address changes to *Psychiatric Clinics of North America*, Elsevier Health Sciences Division, Subscription Customer Service, 3251 Riverport Lane, Maryland Heights, MO 63043. Customer Service: 1-800-654-2452 (US). From outside the United States, call 1-314-447-8871. Fax: 1-314-447-8029. E-mail: journalscustomerservice-usa@elsevier.com (for print support) and journalsonlinesupport-usa@elsevier.com (for online support).

Reprints. For copies of 100 or more, of articles in this publication, please contact the Commercial Reprints Department, Elsevier Inc., 360 Park Avenue South, New York, New York 10010-1710. Tel.: (212) 633-3813, Fax: (212) 462-1935, E-mail: reprints@elsevier.com.

Psychiatric Clinics of North America is covered in *MEDLINE/PubMed (Index Medicus)*, *Current Contents/Social and Behavioral Sciences, Social Science Citation Index, Embase/Excerpta Medica,* and PsycINFO.

Printed and bound by CPI Group (UK) Ltd, Croydon, CR0 4YY

Transferred to digital print 2012

Contributors

EDITORS

CRAIG L. KATZ, MD
Associate Clinical Professor of Psychiatry and Medical Education and Director of the Program in Global Mental Health, Departments of Psychiatry and Medical Education, Icahn School of Medicine at Mount Sinai, New York, New York

ANAND PANDYA, MD
Associate Professor of Clinical Medicine and Vice-Chair for Clinical Affairs, Department of Psychiatry and Behavioral Neurosciences, University of Southern California (USC), Los Angeles, California

AUTHORS

TANJA AUF DER HEYDE, PhD
Department of Psychiatry, Icahn School of Medicine at Mount Sinai, New York, New York

ALI BAHRAMNEJAD, MS, MPH
Mental Health Expert, Kerman University of Medical Sciences, Kerman, Iran

GARY BELKIN, MD, PhD, MPH
Director, Program in Global Mental Health, Associate Professor of Psychiatry, Department of Psychiatry, New York University School of Medicine; Office of Behavioral Health, New York City Health and Hospitals Corporation, New York, New York

FATHER EDDY EUSTACHE, MA
Director, Mental Health, Zanmi Lasante, Cange, Haiti

ALI FARHOUDIAN, MD
Assistant Professor of Psychiatry, Substance Abuse and Dependence Research Center, University of Social Welfare and Rehabilitation Sciences, Tehran, Iran

AHMAD HAJEBI, MD
Assistant Professor of Psychiatry, Department of Psychiatry, Mental Health Research Center, Tehran Psychiatry Institute, Iran University of Medical Sciences, Tehran, Iran

FELICA JONES
Healthy African American Families, Los Angeles, California

CRAIG L. KATZ, MD
Associate Clinical Professor of Psychiatry and Medical Education and Director of the Program in Global Mental Health, Departments of Psychiatry and Medical Education, Icahn School of Medicine at Mount Sinai, New York, New York

ELIZABETH LIZAOLA, MPH
Center for Health Services and Society, Semel Institute for Neuroscience and Human Behavior, University of California, Los Angeles, Los Angeles, California

HOWARD J. OSOFSKY, MD, PhD
Kathleen and John Bricker Chair, Professor and Head, LSU Health Sciences Center, Department of Psychiatry, New Orleans, Louisiana

JOY D. OSOFSKY, PhD
Barbara Lemann Professor, Departments of Pediatrics and Psychiatry, LSU Health Sciences Center, New Orleans, Louisiana

CATE OSWALD, MPH
Director of Haiti Programs, Partners In Health, Boston, Massachusetts

FATIH OZBAY, MD
Medical Director, The WTC Mental Health Program; Departments of Psychiatry and Preventive Medicine, Icahn School of Medicine at Mount Sinai, New York, New York

ALONZO PLOUGH, PhD, MPH
Emergency Preparedness and Response, Los Angeles County Department of Public Health, Los Angeles, California

GIUSEPPE RAVIOLA, MD, MPH
Director, Program in Global Mental Health and Social Change, Assistant Professor of Psychiatry, and Global Heath and Social Medicine, Departments of Psychiatry, and Global Health and Social Medicine, Harvard Medical School; Director, Mental Health, Partners In Health; Director, Psychiatry Quality Program, Boston Children's Hospital, Boston, Massachusetts

DORI REISSMAN, MD
Medical Director, The WTC Health Program, National Institute for Occupational Health and Safety, Centers for Disease Control and Prevention, Atlanta, Georgia

G. JAMES RUBIN, PGCAP, MSc, PhD
Department of Psychological Medicine, Weston Education Centre, King's College London, London, United Kingdom

JENNIFER SEVERE, MD
Dr Mario Pagenel Fellow in Global Mental Health Delivery, Partners In Health, Harvard Medical School, Boston, Massachusetts; Zanmi Lasante, Cange, Haiti

SANDIP SHAH, MD
Research Director and Professor of Psychiatry, Department of Psychiatry, SBKS MI & RC, Sumandeep Vidyapeeth, Vadodara, India

VANSH SHARMA, MD
Department of Psychiatry, Icahn School of Medicine at Mount Sinai, New York, New York

JUN SHIGEMURA, MD, PhD
Department of Psychiatry, National Defense Medical College, Saitama, Japan

DAYA SOMASUNDARAM, MD, FRCPsych, FRANZCP, FSLCP
Professor, Department of Psychiatry, University of Jaffna, Jaffna, Sri Lanka; University of Adelaide, Australia

BENJAMIN F. SPRINGGATE, MD, MPH
RAND Health, RAND Corporation, Santa Monica, California

TATIANA THEROSME, BA
Zanmi Lasante, Cange, Haiti

KENNETH B. WELLS, MD, MPH
Center for Health Services and Society, Semel Institute for Neuroscience and Human Behavior; Department of Health Services, School of Public Health, University of California, Los Angeles, Los Angeles, California; RAND Health, RAND Corporation, Santa Monica, California

SIMON WESSELY, MA, BM, BCh, MSc, MD, FRCP, FRCPsych, FMedSci, FKC
Department of Psychological Medicine, Weston Education Centre, King's College London, London, United Kingdom

JUN YAMASHITA, PhD
Faculty of Letters, Department of Humanities and Social Sciences, Keio University, Tokyo, Japan

Contents

health approach was implemented by providing a common room in temporary housing developments to build a sense of community and to approach evacuees so that they could be triaged and referred to mental health teams. Japan now advocates using psychological first aid to educate first responders. This article extracts key lessons from relevant literature.

Education and training about immediate responses are important for all mental health providers of immediate and continuing services to assist children, adolescents, adults, and families in the aftermath of disasters. To sensitively help with evacuations and return to normalcy, responders must also be trained to understand the culture and traditions of affected communities. It is important to provide knowledge about available resources and to emphasize the need for routines and self-care for both victims and responders in an environment that, with recovery, will reflect a new normal.

The 2003 Bam earthquake was one of the most catastrophic disasters to have struck Iran. This article summarizes the short-term and long-term psychological, social, and economic impacts of the Bam earthquake on survivors across a decade since its occurrence. Identification and definition of capability as well as recognizing the nature and extent of personal and social capabilities in a community are priceless in preventing disasters and reducing their consequent destruction.

This report emphasizes the belief that whatever the type and scale of disaster, the period of transition from relief to recovery is the most critical. Following the severe earthquake that struck Kachchh, Gurjarat, India on 26 January 2001, emotions spanned grief over the lives lost; anxiety over property and other economic losses; profound feelings of isolation, helplessness, and guilt; and panic in the face of problematic communications from authorities. In an attempt to manage this vast array of psychosocial problems, a large cadre of volunteers was rapidly trained and supervised by experts to work as grass-roots counselors for the community.

The authors review the existing literature on the mental health impact of the September 11th attacks and the implications for disaster mental health clinicians and policy makers. The authors discuss the demographic characteristics of those affected and the state of mental health needs and existing mental health delivery services; the nature of the disaster and primary impacts on lives, infrastructure, and socioeconomic factors; the acute aftermath in the days and weeks after the attacks; the persistent mental health impact and evolution of services of the postacute aftermath; and the implications for future disaster mental health practitioners and policy makers.

This article presents an overview of the mental health response to the 2010 Haiti earthquake. Discussion includes consideration of complexities that relate to emergency response, mental health and psychosocial response in disasters, long-term planning of systems of care, and the development of safe, effective, and culturally sound mental health services in the Haitian context. This information will be of value to mental health professionals and policy specialists interested in mental health in Haiti, and in the delivery of mental health services in particularly resource-limited contexts in the setting of disasters.

Awareness of the impact of disasters globally on mental health is increasing. Known difficulties in preparing communities for disasters and a lack of focus on relationship building and organizational capacity in preparedness and response have led to a greater policy focus on community resiliency as a key public health approach to disaster response. In this article, the authors describe how an approach to community engagement for improving mental health services, disaster recovery, and preparedness from a community resiliency perspective emerged from their work in applying a partnered, participatory research framework, iteratively, in Los Angeles County and the City of New Orleans.

PSYCHIATRIC CLINICS OF NORTH AMERICA

FORTHCOMING ISSUES

Late Life Depression
W. Vaughn McCall, MD, *Editor*

Neuropsychiatry of Traumatic Brain Injury
Ricardo Jorge, MD, and
David Arciniegas, MD, *Editors*

Obsessive Compulsive and Related Disorders
Wayne Goodman, MD, *Editor*

RECENT ISSUES

June 2013
Psychiatric Manifestations of Neurotoxins
Daniel E. Rusyniak, MD, and
Michael R. Dobbs, MD, *Editors*

March 2013
Complementary and Integrative Therapies for Psychiatric Disorders
Philip R. Muskin, MD,
Patricia L. Gerbarg, MD, and
Richard P. Brown, MD, *Editors*

December 2012
Forensic Psychiatry
Charles L. Scott, MD, *Editor*

RELATED INTEREST

Psychiatry Research
30 June 2013 (Vol. 208, No. 1)
Face it: Collecting mental health and disaster related data using Facebook vs. personal interview: The case of the 2011 Fukushima nuclear disaster
Menachem Ben-Ezra, Yuval Palgi, Or Aviel, et al.

DOWNLOAD
Free App!

Review Articles
THE CLINICS

NOW AVAILABLE FOR YOUR iPhone and iPad

Preface

Disasters: A Global Perspective

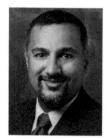 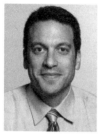

Anand Pandya, MD   Craig L. Katz, MD
Editors

Although disasters are tragically too common, they are infrequent enough so that most psychiatrists who respond to disasters will do so only once or twice over the course of their careers. Thus they may have difficulty separating aspects that are unique to a single disaster from issues that are more universal in disaster psychiatry. This challenge is reflected in the disaster psychiatry literature whereby many articles and books provide deep insights into a single disaster but do not help the reader understand what is inherent to the field of disaster psychiatry.

We, the guest editors of this issue, may have fallen into this trap in our writings over the years. Shortly after the September 11 attacks, we began planning a volume of *Psychiatric Clinics of North America* focused on disaster psychiatry. Although that volume provided a broad perspective on different aspects of the field, almost all of the authors were from the United States and their research and clinical expertise derived primarily from American disasters.

For all of the shock that met the Boston Marathon bombing earlier this year, those events unfolded in front of a nation and a field that was far more aware of the possibility of terrorism and other disasters than we were at the time of the September 11 attacks. The dramatic pursuit of the Tsarnaev brothers in the days that followed prolonged the period before the residents of the Boston area could consider this threat from any distance and yet the relatively rapid, coordinated response demonstrates how the United States has changed after a decade-long focus on preparedness.

The current volume benefits from this decade of heightened awareness of context and we hope to correct some of our earlier myopia by placing disasters in a global context. Except for an article by Dr Ken Wells that compares disaster preparedness in 2 different cities, each of the articles in this volume represents different disasters from around the world. To minimize the risk of skewing the view through an outsider's lens, almost all the authors have had long-standing relationships with the mental health systems in the area of the disaster. One exception is our first-person account by C.L.K. describing his work in El Salvador, where he was very much an outsider.

Psychiatr Clin N Am 36 (2013) xi–xii
http://dx.doi.org/10.1016/j.psc.2013.05.007
0193-953X/13/$ – see front matter © 2013 Published by Elsevier Inc.

We hope that this personal narrative will provide a human-scale view to counterbalance the usual view from 10,000 feet needed to describe the impact of disasters on a society and the large-scale interventions that follow.

Each author was asked to contextualize disaster psychiatry beyond the acute stage of the disaster, looking at both the pre-event society and the long-term psychological and social trajectory of the postevent society—typically, a marathon of its own kind. The results offer a rich opportunity to appreciate the broad range of work that falls under disaster psychiatry. The predisaster mental health services in Haiti stand in striking contrast to those in London so it is not surprising that the postdisaster work will vary also. Disaster psychiatrists in Haiti focused on developing the most basic level of mental health services, while those in London were able to rapidly conduct more systematic research about how individuals respond to disasters and the effectiveness of specific postdisaster mental health interventions.

If psychiatry can provide a unique contribution to future disaster responses, it will be based on our ability to step back from single case studies to an examination of larger patterns. We hope that this volume helps the field to take a step in that direction.

We very much thank Elsevier and our editor, Joanne Husovski, for giving us the platform to take another, hopefully wiser, look at disaster psychiatry.

Anand Pandya, MD
Department of Psychiatry & Behavioral Neurosciences
University of Southern California (USC)
Los Angeles, CA 90089, USA

Craig L. Katz, MD
Program in Global Mental Health &
the Departments of Psychiatry and Medical Education
Icahn School of Medicine at Mount Sinai
New York, NY 10029, USA

E-mail addresses:
anandpandya@hotmail.com (A. Pandya)
craig.katz@mssm.edu (C.L. Katz)

First Person
A Mental Health Mission to Post-Earthquake El Salvador

Craig L. Katz, MD

KEYWORDS

• El Salvador earthquake • Disaster psychiatry • Post-disaster outreach

KEY POINTS

- Disaster related mental health issues unfold over months to years.
- Disaster mental health services should occur in the context of the pre-event state of the community.
- Disaster mental health care must be sustainable beyond the acute phase of a disaster.
- Collaboration with medical services is essential to effective disaster mental health outreach.

In February 2001, 3 psychiatrists flew from New York City to assist survivors of a major earthquake in El Salvador. As the head of Disaster Psychiatry Outreach (DPO), a 2-year-old nonprofit organization devoted to utilizing the expertise and goodwill of psychiatrists to help disaster-stricken communities, I spearheaded and led the mission. As written about previously by Lynn Delisi, my senior colleague on that trip, it was among our organization's earliest responses and our, and my, first internationally.[1] We got by with our collective will and intuition.

It is hard to know when a disaster ends, given the myriad strands it entails and the many peoples and places affected. Indeed, it has been suggested that where human recovery takes about 10 times longer than infrastructure recovery, psychological recovery in particular takes incalculably longer.[2] We were in El Salvador for exactly 2 weeks and, knowing that mental health needs related to the earthquake would not abate according to our travel plans, we promised to be back and, as so many people begged of us, not to forget about them.

We did keep our promise and a different group of us returned in May 2002, still trying to ascertain how we could possibly make a long-term difference in a place with so few mental health resources and so many needs, whether earthquake related or not. That trip launched the idea of working with a children's museum in San Salvador, the Tin Marin Museum, as a platform to reach children traumatized by the earthquake, prior civil war, abundant gangs, domestic violence, or poverty. Two more trips in 2005

Departments of Psychiatry and Medical Education, Icahn School of Medicine at Mount Sinai, Box 1257, New York, NY 10029, USA
E-mail address: craig.katz@mssm.edu

Psychiatr Clin N Am 36 (2013) 309–319
http://dx.doi.org/10.1016/j.psc.2013.05.005
0193-953X/13/$ – see front matter © 2013 Elsevier Inc. All rights reserved.

and then 2009 have so far yielded research data about knowledge of and attitudes toward sexual abuse, but no new services.

We do not know when, or even if, we will return to El Salvador. Nor have the fits and starts of our trips yet coalesced into a cohesive narrative about the long-term mental health aftermath of the 2001 earthquake. In fact, when I asked a Salvadoran colleague and friend whom I met at the Tin Marin museum if he could provide that narrative for this issue, he said he was not aware that such a story existed or could readily be written from even from his own perch in San Salvador.

Fortuitously, I recently rediscovered my journal (**Fig. 1**) from our 2001 trip to El Salvador. Leafing through the scrawl contained in that blue spiral notebook, I realized it does provide a long-term perspective in its own right. It permits a look back through the prism of more than a decade of subsequent disaster and international experiences in psychiatry that my colleagues and I have gone on to amass via DPO. In the nascent wisdom of that journal lie some invaluable pearls about disasters and mental health.

In what follows, I excerpt and discuss salient quotes or moments from the journal. The reader is encouraged to see how much of it applies, or not, to the stories and ideas shared by the many contributors to this issue. Indeed, it will be difficult not to reference some of the articles and the events they cover in this retrospective.

BACKGROUND

El Salvador today, with its population of 6,090,646 and life expectancy of 73.69 years, is the third largest economy in Central America. The economy rests largely on agriculture and industry, and 36.5% of Salvadorans live below the poverty line.[3] El Salvador ranked 105 out of 187 countries in the 2011 Human Development Index.[4]

The earthquake that struck El Salvador on January 13, 2001 registered 7.6 on the Richter Scale, with the epicenter offshore in the Pacific Ocean (**Fig. 2**). At least 944

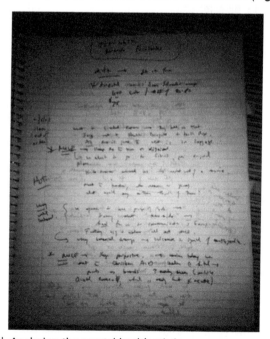

Fig. 1. The journal. Analyzing the mental health mission.

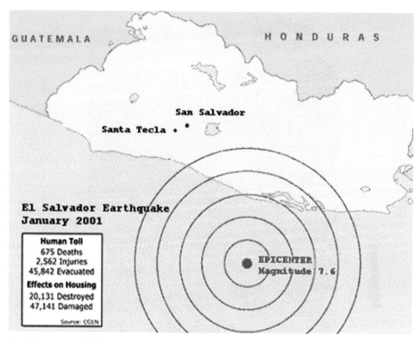

GUATEMALA

HONDURAS

San Salvador

Santa Tecla •

El Salvador Earthquake January 2001

Human Toll
675 Deaths
2,562 Injuries
45,842 Evacuated
Effects on Housing
20,131 Destroyed
47,141 Damaged
Source: CCEN

EPICENTER
Magnitude 7.6

Fig. 2. Epicenter of El Salvador earthquake.

people were killed, 5565 injured, 108,261 houses destroyed, 169,692 houses damaged, and more than 150,000 buildings damaged (**Fig. 3**) in El Salvador.[5]

We traveled to El Salvador with a larger team of medical professionals from the American Jewish World Service (AJWS) several weeks later, from February 3 to February 16, 2001. On the ground, we worked with AJWS's local partner, La Coordinadora, as well as several agencies we met in the country.

February 4

Is it necessary to live like a victim to help victims?

One of the earliest notations in the journal came after our first night in El Salvador and was written in Ciudad Romero, a rural town where La Coordinadora was headquartered. We had been left to stay overnight in the town's community center, with no beds, working phones, running water, or provisions (**Fig. 4**). We had come prepared but not that prepared; we were miserable waiting for our hosts to arrive on a Sunday morning when no one was in sight and everyone must have been in church. When they finally did, we undiplomatically insisted they take us back to San Salvador, where we paid out of pocket to put ourselves up in a hotel for the rest of the trip.

In fact, some of us were better prepared for the vagaries and inconveniences of disaster relief and international travel than others, which is something I have seen over and over since then: not every mental health professional is suited to pursuing disaster work. It is critical that any psychiatrist or mental health professional who chooses to work in a disaster-affected community (when disaster affects one's own community, there is less choice) ask themselves about their motivations, their goals, and their personal and professional readiness. In truth, any worthy relief agency

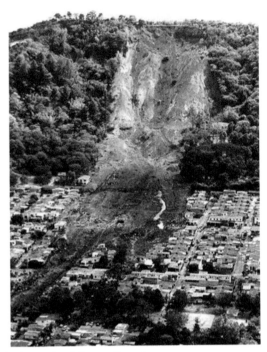

Fig. 3. The physical aftermath of the earthquake.

should be asking, and answering, the same questions of its volunteers. I have learned that some psychiatrists can do just as much good by staying in their usual work and "holding down the fort" while others deploy to disaster-stricken communities to help.

Readers of this issue might even consider what made them decide to read it in the first place and what they imagine, literally, they will do with what they learn.

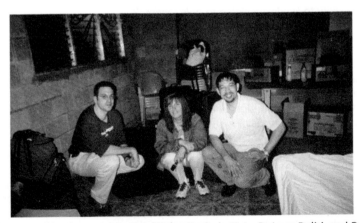

Fig. 4. Three psychiatrists arrive in El Salvador. Dr Craig Katz, Dr Lynn Delisi, and Dr Enrique Villareal in the community center living accommodations.

February 5

Our first activity is a visit to a "medical brigade."

It is telling that our first clinical activity in El Salvador involved traveling with mobile clinics that drove around to villages providing basic medical care (**Fig. 5**), both pre- and post-earthquake. For multiple reasons, they did not usually incorporate mental health care. Later on February 14 at another medical brigade, I went on to write, "I just walk around and talk with families—lots of somatic complaints—headache, foot pain, chest pain, and so forth—did not emphasize emotions."

In so many places in the world, even in psychiatry-rich urban settings in the developed world, people in distress are much more likely to present complaining of physical aches and pains than emotional suffering. These pains may arise from medical or psychiatric origins, and medical sequelae of disasters predispose to comorbid mental health issues. Amid all of the tangible concerns in the postdisaster environment, this is even more so the case. Psychiatrists intending to help postdisaster communities should give consideration to colocating their services with their medical colleagues. This enables more readily accessed services to make mental health referrals, and for the psychiatrist to help sort out where physical distress ends and emotional distress begins in a population at risk for the latter.

The World Trade Center Mental Health Program described by Ozbay and colleagues in this issue, with its integration of mental health screenings and treatment into the medical screenings and treatment of 9/11 responders, embodies this more than I ever could have envisioned back in 2001 in El Salvador, some 8 months before the 9/11 attacks occurred.

February 5–6

Talk with some people but where to start? Need food and shelter...

As we got to know members of other relief agencies staying at our San Salvador hotel, we learned about San Augustine, a rural town reputed to have been especially devastated by the earthquake. It was suggested that the mental health problems there must

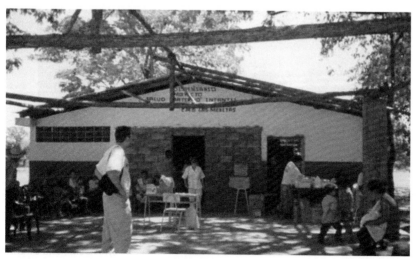

Fig. 5. El Salvador village medical clinic after the earthquake.

be especially acute, leading us to visit this town later on February 5, ready to evaluate townspeople with mental health surveys we had brought (**Fig. 6**).

In fact, we found a town that seemed flattened by some unearthly force and that had somehow been neglected by most relief agencies. Before we could unfurl our surveys, we were struck by how the people of San Augustine needed basics such as food and water. We decided to drive back to San Salvador, where we purchased rice, beans, portable heating kits, and water, and returned the next day to distribute them (**Fig. 7**).

Although we were ill-equipped and untrained to be doing food distribution, we did our best by doing what seemed humane. We would have been a parody of psychiatric selves to have been asking the community members the iconic question of our profession, "how are you?," when they had empty bellies. In this way, we anticipated the framework known as Psychological First Aid (PFA) that was promulgated after 9/11, which emphasizes addressing people's basic physical and human needs as a means to help them feel better before turning to traditional psychiatric interventions such as psychotherapy and medications.[6]

The reader will see PFA referenced at different points in this issue in countries as far from El Salvador as 3/11-affected Japan. Although PFA is traditionally thought of as guiding interventions in the acute aftermath of a disaster, it is worth thinking about its message of basics first over the long term. For example, how does one conceive of mental health in the 3/11-affected region of northern Japan when people displaced by the radiation released by the tsunami still find themselves living in temporary housing and in places far from their homes nearly 2 years later?

February 7

> Meet with psychiatrist from Health Ministry—afraid that people are not being detected with mental illness. But, also not sure what he would do if they all came.

This conversation took place in El Cafetalon, a soccer field that was transformed into an evacuation camp (**Fig. 8**) for 3500 people scattered by the earthquake and mudslides in a suburb of the capital known as New San Salvador. As eager as we were to deploy our mental health surveys in the name of finding suffering

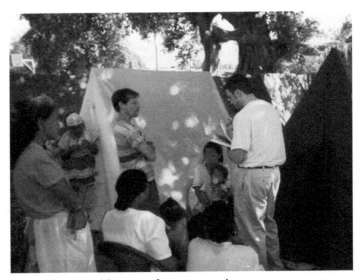

Fig. 6. The outreach team with surveys for town members.

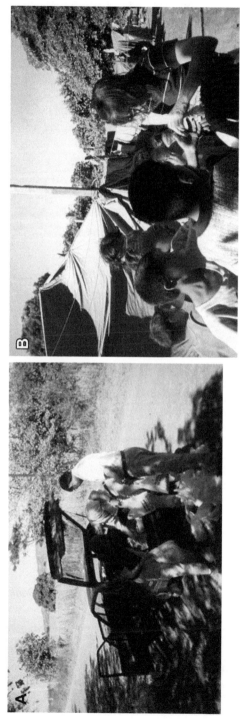

Fig. 7. (A) The Basics - The outreach team readies for distribution of water and food. (B) The outreach team distributes the supplies amid chaos.

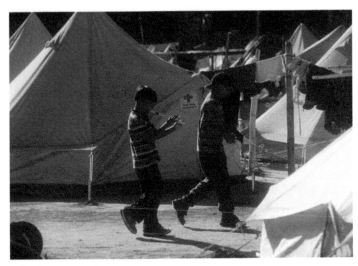

Fig. 8. El Cafetalon evacuation camp.

in the dimpled sea of white tents, we did not have a ready answer for our Salvadoran colleague's concern about the chronic shortage of mental health professionals in his country.

We belatedly would come across the answer when we responded in 2005 to post-tsunami Sri Lanka. There we wound up partnering with a local mental health nonprofit organization in remote northeastern Sri Lanka known as Annai Illam. Under the direction of Father Edmund Reginald, a Jesuit priest with a Masters in Psychology, nearly 2 dozen lay mental health counselors with no more than the equivalent of a high school education had been trained to offer basic psychotherapy services to assist people affected by that country's then civil war as well as the eventual tsunami. "Father Reggie" took local human resources and maximized their potential and, surely, there was a way for our colleague to do the same at El Cafetalon. In 2010, DPO would likewise provide Haitian nursing students with basic mental health training they otherwise lacked in order for them to help their country recover from an earthquake. Maybe our Salvadoran colleague could even have trained otherwise idle residents of the camp to provide basic psychotherapy services to their neighbors, an approach that has even since been written about in literature from Uganda.[7]

Throughout this issue are many other worldwide examples of how to put local resources to work in the name of mental health.

February 9

Snake in the river causes it [the earthquake]...Afraid Central America will disappear.

We leave as rumors re: volcano circulate and as people line up for food—Jane is 'freaking out.'

In 2 different Salvadoran towns, Ciudad Romero and San Miguel, and in 1 day, we were inexplicably confronted by dire rumors and enough fear to unnerve at least one of my fellow travelers. It is tempting to look at fears of all-powerful river snakes and long-dormant volcanoes as the product of poor education, naïveté, and parochial living. But in disaster after disaster, in many places, we have found that a mythology inevitably arises through which a stricken community both seeks to find explanations and to localize their fears.

On our 2005 post-tsunami mission to Sri Lanka, we came upon a large blackboard on which a fantastical picture of a monstrous sky and ocean were drawn below a caption in Tamil: "Tsunami: real or imagined?" (**Fig. 9**).

In post-9/11 New York, fears about the potentially cancerous effects of the dust and other substances at Ground Zero continue to abound today even as scientists have yet to find clear evidence to substantiate these concerns.[8]

Every article in this issue exemplifies how different communities and countries try to make sense of things even as they try to make order, spanning the dust of Ground Zero to the radiologic contamination of Fukushima, Japan.

February 13

Always keep medical equipment with you. You NEVER know.

While driving to the psychiatric hospital in San Salvador to better educate ourselves about the range of local mental health services, the car in which we were driving began to swerve. I soon realized this was not reckless driving but rather another earthquake that reached 6.6 on the Richter scale. When things were still and we learned on the car radio that the town of San Vincente outside of San Salvador was especially devastated, including the collapse of a school, we rushed to help in any way we could.

We were admitted into the swirling scene at the main hospital in San Vincente when we identified ourselves as physicians. Unfortunately, we had left all of our medical equipment, such as stethoscopes and antibiotics brought by our pediatric colleague, at the hotel. We made do, borrowing equipment and providing pediatric and medical care to the extent that each of us was comfortable (**Fig. 10**). We also helped patients who had been evacuated from the hospital to an outdoor courtyard under the unrelenting sun to make room for the newly wounded. Without cups, we filled latex gloves with water and squeezed it via pinpricks in the fingertips of the glove into the thirsty mouths of patients lying around.

This was not the time for psychiatry as we normally know it and practice it. Again echoing the de facto practice of PFA in San Augustine, what we tried to do was meet more basic needs for medical care and nurturance. The ideal disaster mental health professional is someone who sees himself or herself as a humanitarian first, a physician second, and a psychiatrist third. That is the posture and practice required

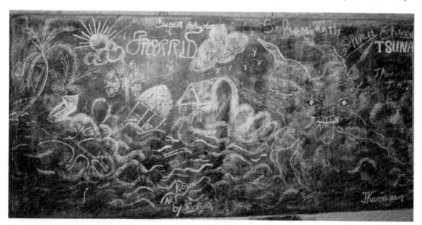

Fig. 9. Blackboard drawing of tsunami in Sri Lanka.

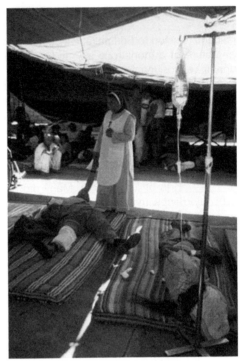

Fig. 10. In San Vincente, acute medical needs preceded psychiatric needs.

to best integrate mental health professionals into disaster response, especially in the impact and acute phase of a disaster (**Fig. 11**). And, over the long term that is the focus of this issue, a psychiatrist likely heals best when the hierarchy of human needs is remembered.

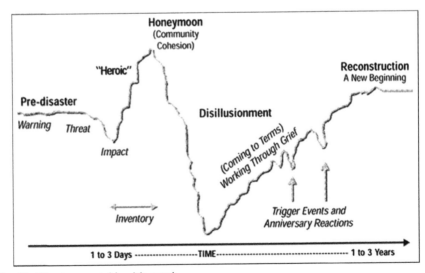

Fig. 11. Disaster mental health graph.

February 16

There is so much that has happened to us. Not just the earthquake.

Thus intoned a community health worker on our last day in El Salvador in the town of Ciudad Romero where we began our trip. Thinking about the prior civil war and past epidemics, they were explaining why it was important that we not forget them even as the acuity of the earthquake passed. This quote is a fitting one on which to end this article, as this issue really is very much about how different places and different people have found the will and the way to address long-term mental health issues long after the real and figurative dust has settled on their disaster-affected communities. As a sign in a US Government relief agency's office in Sri Lanka so accurately stated, "It's a marathon, not a sprint."

REFERENCES

1. Delisi L. Aftermath of earthquake in El Salvador. In: Pandya A, Katz C, editors. Disaster psychiatry: intervening when nightmares come true. Hillsdale (NJ): The Analytic Press; 2004. p. 133–44.
2. Chandra A, Acosta J. Disaster recovery also involves human recovery. J Am Med Assoc 2010;14:1608–9.
3. The human development index. 2011. Available at: http://hdr.undp.org/en. Accessed September 30, 2012.
4. CIA world factbook. 2012. Available at: www.cia.gov. Accessed September 30, 2012.
5. 2001 El Salvador earthquakes. Available at: https://en.wikipedia.org/wiki/2001_El_Salvador_earthquakes. Accessed May 15, 2013.
6. Psychological first aid—field operations guide. 2nd edition. Available at: http://www.ptsd.va.gov/professional/manuals/psych-first-aid.asp. Accessed May 15, 2013.
7. Neuner F, Lamaro Onyut P. Treatment of posttraumatic stress disorder by trained lay counselors in an African refugee settlement: a randomized controlled trial. J Consult Clin Psychol 2008;76:686–94.
8. Li J, Cone J, Kahn AR, et al. Association between World Trade Center exposure and excess cancer risk. J Am Med Assoc 2012;308(23):2479–88.

Recent Disasters in Sri Lanka
Lessons Learned

Daya Somasundaram, MD, FRCPsych, FRANZCP, FSLCP[a,b,]*

KEYWORDS

- Disaster • War • Tsunami • Collective trauma • Community approaches

KEY POINTS

- It is worthwhile planning beforehand to prevent or mitigate the impact of disasters at the community and family levels.
- There should be regional and international mechanisms to protect civilians in times of conflict or when powerful leaders and states overstep boundaries of good governance and observation of basic rights.
- In the long-term, there is a need to create a culture of peace by social peace building.

BACKGROUND: SRI LANKAN SOCIETY BEFORE CONFLICT AND NATURAL DISASTER

Sri Lanka, a small island off the southern tip of India, has faced devastating disasters, both artificial and natural, in the recent past. Sri Lanka is a resource-poor, low-income developing country that has been struggling socioeconomically and politically to keep its head above water. However, the country has not always been this way, and recent history has important lessons to teach on how particular development trajectories can make countries and populations vulnerable to disasters. Man-made disasters like war can be prevented by conflict resolution strategies, and the impact of most natural disasters can be mitigated by appropriate planning and preparedness. It became clear in responding to the major disasters that widespread mental health and psychosocial consequences can best be addressed by appropriate public mental health measures.

Although Ceylon, as Sri Lanka was then called, received her independence from Britain in 1948 on a sound economic footing with a large sterling balance and well-developed plantation sector, world trends were not favorable. Belatedly, there was some diversification of her foreign exchange earnings with garments, tourism, and

Disclosures: No conflict of interest.
[a] Department of Psychiatry, University of Jaffna, Jaffna, Sri Lanka; [b] University of Adelaide, Adelaide, South Australia
* Corresponding author. Department of Psychiatry, University of Jaffna, Jaffna, Sri Lanka.
E-mail address: manathu@gmail.com

Psychiatr Clin N Am 36 (2013) 321–338
http://dx.doi.org/10.1016/j.psc.2013.05.001
0193-953X/13/$ – see front matter © 2013 Elsevier Inc. All rights reserved.

sending workers mainly to the Middle East, who remitted their wages. Lanka lacked easily exploitable natural resources. There continued to be heavy spending on welfare measures like health, education, social benefits, and subsidies to agriculture, rice, state-run institutions, and state ventures increasingly funded by foreign aid and loans. With the dramatic decrease in death rates from control of malaria, use of antibiotics, and improvements in medical health care, the population increased geometrically. The population density, particularly in the crowded southwest of the country, reached uncomfortable proportions for a small island nation, which made people naturally look for less populated areas. The tragedy for modern Lanka has been that it never produced a great statesman like a Nehru, Gandhi, or Mandela who could rise above petty sectarian differences and act for the national interest, to plan and lead the country to the much-coveted Newly Industrialized Country status. Instead, the country descended into bitter interparty feuding, with the two national parties using all their ingenuity and skills to come in to and stay in power. The democratic system implanted by Britain did not thrive, unlike in neighboring India. Increasingly, each election (both before, during, and after the election) became an orgy of threats, abduction, and killing of opposition candidates and their supporters; voter intimidation, rigging, ballot stuffing, impersonation, obstruction, and destruction of booths followed by violence by the victors against the losers (post-election curfew is routine practice). The goal was to win by any means possible and then stay in power. The charade of democracy, which none of the elite seemed to believe in, was enacted at election times for external and internal consumption. With more close election monitoring by national and international bodies, the level of violence has at least declined. On the positive side, there have been periodic elections with a parliament (although with decreasing power because of the introduction of an authoritarian presidential system, in which most of the ministers are given lucrative cabinet posts, attracting many in the opposition to cross over), press, judiciary, police, local government, and various committees even at institutional and organizational levels. However, the usual checks and balances that characterize democracy, the give-and-take of negotiations, debate and discussions, and the impartial rule of law have proved illusory. There is no real division of power between the executive, legislature, and judiciary. Gradually, particularly after the 1970s and the introduction of the presidential system, these powers became concentrated at the top, in the head of state. The freedom and independence of the press were gradually muzzled. Many of the more able journalists left the country, were killed, or were made to fall silent. The current press has become polarized and inflammatory, aggravating and engendering ethnic passions. The justice system has been cowed into partiality, silence and favoritism.[1,2] More importantly, Lanka lacked the tradition and practice of democratic institutions, civil organizations, public discourse, respect and belief systems, and protection of civil liberties and minority rights that would have allowed democracy to function. The temptation behind the democratic façade had always been toward authoritarianism, with absolute, dictatorial control, much like the old feudal kings.[3] Corruption,[4] a close nexus between politicians and the criminal underworld, nepotism and clientism or patronage, by which stalwarts and loyalists were rewarded with jobs and influence in the bloated, inefficient state sector,[5] and short-sighted, poor planning led the country to economic ruin, to the brink of becoming a failed state. The historic exclusion from governance and access to state resources and opportunities for the disgruntled rural and urban educated Sinhala youth in the south led to two Janatha Vimukthi Perumana (JVP) uprisings or manmade disasters in the 1970s and late 1980s.[6] The state responded with the full might of its repressive apparatus with the help of India and other countries. The death toll in the second blood letting was variously estimated to be more than 60,000, with daily reports of disappearances, of men being dragged from their families in the dead of night to be tortured and killed and their bodies destroyed on makeshift pyres of old tires (Derek Brown, *Manchester Guardian*, December 15, 1988). The same methods of repressive measures were then used by the state to squash the ethnic rebellion in the north and east.

Within the global trend since the end of World War II of increasing intrastate, ethnic civil wars,[7,8] Sri Lanka is often studied as one of the examples of ethnic conflict that progressed to war,[7,9–15] with a casualty list of more than 100,000 killed, and many more injured, mentally affected, displaced both internally and overseas, and communities, property, and ecosystems destroyed.[16] Although the physical fighting drew to a close in May, 2009, it is pertinent to look at what caused the conflict and its psychosocial consequences to communities, because the underlying issues remain unresolved. Further, an understanding of what happened in Lanka helps shed light on similar contexts and dynamics elsewhere in the world and perhaps can lead to measures to prevent manmade disasters. After gaining independence in a postcolonial context, the Sinhala ruling elite representing the majority were unwilling to build a broad-based multicultural politics; the big power rivalry, economic interests, and the competition for jobs and resources could have played itself out in healthier ways, as in India,[17] if the politics had not been shaped so strongly by exclusive nationalistic ideologies that created horizontal inequities.[18] European theories of race, largely discredited by the early twentieth century, gave rise to virulent ideologies (Sinhala and its mirror image, Tamil), which have driven the ethnic conflict.

Although the health sector had been well developed and health care was free, mental health care continued to be neglected. Centralized care around the capital, Colombo, was available in a few archaic asylum like institutions, with few mental health professionals. Treatment approaches were mainly drug oriented for major psychotic disorders. There had been some belated efforts at decentralization, and limited mental health services were functioning at the district levels when the disasters struck. These systems were grossly inadequate to meet the sudden demands of major disasters and did not possess the multidisciplinary teams or the public mental health reach to deal with the large populations affected.

RECENT DISASTERS
Manmade Disaster: War

The Sri Lankan state, the various Tamil militants, in particular the Liberation Tigers of Tamil Eelam (LTTE, which for more than two decades fought to create a separate state), the Sinhala JVP (an ultraleftist militant group that made two attempts violently to overthrow the government), and India (during its short intervention in the island [1987–90] to impose peace), were all involved in a dirty war,[19,20] with grave human rights violations and crimes against humanity.[6,21] Critical at times, the international community, its many organizations, diplomatic missions, the United Nations (UN), and aid agencies giving technical support, military hardware, training, and the global network of socioeconomic ties and mutual relationships that give covert recognition, legitimacy, and tacit sanction as well as the Sri Lankan and Tamil diaspora communities that supported the conflict were also indirectly implicated.[19,20,22] Although the physical fighting ended dramatically in the Vanni in May, 2009, with the state using indiscriminate shelling and bombing as the LTTE held the civilian population hostage that resulted in more than 40,000 civilians deaths, many more injuries, and unacknowledged war crimes,[22–28] the underlying ethnocentrism and political causes remain unresolved.

Natural Disaster: Asian Tsunami of 2004

The gigantic Asian tsunami of December 26, 2004 was generated by one of the worst earthquakes on record, measuring 9 on the Richter scale, with an epicenter just off the coast in Aceh, Indonesia (**Fig. 1**).

A series of massive tidal waves sped across the Indian Ocean, killing more than 220,000 people in 12 countries spanning Southeast Asia, South Asia, and East Africa, and displaced more than 1.6 million people in addition to colossal property and infrastructure damage. In Sri Lanka, more than a million of its people were affected; the tsunami displaced more than 800,000 people, destroyed their homes and belongings, and killed 36,000 from the coastal communities of the northeast and south (**Fig. 2**).[29] Ninety percent of those killed were from the fishing community and belonged to the lower socioeconomic class.[30]

The suddenness and massive nature of the wave(s) overwhelmed and shocked everyone. The deaths, injuries, destruction, and chaos were unprecedented. Poignantly affected was the strong organic bond and intimate relationship that the coastal community, many of them fisher folks, had with the sea. Most depended on the sea for their livelihood and had grown up in the coastal environment of the sea. The rupturing of the organic bond and the fear for the sea would take time to heal. Many could not face the sea in the immediate aftermath and would not venture near the coast. The songs, the poems, drawings, narratives, and dramas from that time reflected this deep agony that was caused by the tsunami.

The World Health Organization (WHO) estimated that 30% to 50% of those affected were at risk of developing psychological distress or mental health problems needing help and support, whereas 5% to 10% would develop severe problems (such as pathologic grief, posttraumatic stress disorder [PTSD], and depression), needing specific intervention and treatment.[31] There was an immediate and generous local response, in which people from all communities came forward to help those affected with support, shelter, clothing, and food. People from different ethnic communities (Sinhala, Tamil, Muslim and others), from different religions

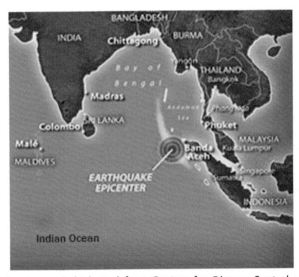

Fig. 1. 2004 Asian tsunami. (*Adapted from* Centers for Disease Control and Prevention. Available at: http://www.cdc.gov/bam/safety/tsunami-where.html; Accessed July 23, 2013.)

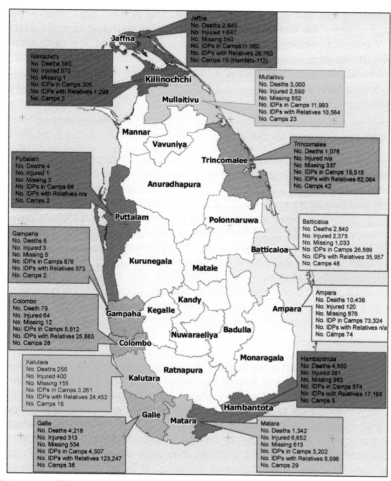

Fig. 2. Impact of the tsunami on Sri Lanka. (*Courtesy of* Center for National Operations (CNO), Govt of Sri Lanka, Colombo. The CNO was created to manage the Post-Tsunami recovery programme and has since been officially closed. The figure is used with the permission of the Director, CNO.)

(Buddhist, Hindu and Muslim), different castes, ages and walks of life (military, militants, political parties, and ordinary folks) helped each other naturally and warmly without barriers, animosity, or prejudice. There was a feeling of social solidarity, cohesion, and camaraderie. For a brief moment, there was hope that the tsunami had brought together the ethnic groups and healed the strife and conflict. There was also an unprecedented massive international humanitarian response of sympathy, aid and personnel, which poured into the country. A whole culture of non-governmental organizations (NGOs) developed around the tsunami rehabilitation work,[31,32] which at times became overwhelming, taking on a carnival atmosphere.[33] The state response was tardy and discriminatory, marked by politics, favoritism, and corruption.[31,34,35]

The tsunami accentuated rather than ameliorated the conflict dynamics. In spite of initial hopes that the tsunami response would provide a space to re-energize peace negotiations, it had the opposite effect, deepening political fault lines. Protracted negotiations about the institutional arrangements for delivering tsunami assistance to the North-East mirrored earlier peace talks and exposed the deep underlying problems of flawed governance, entrenched positions, and patronage politics.[35]

The pre-disaster social conditions in northern Sri Lanka and the impact of the manmade and natural disasters, although they had many similarities, also had important differences (**Table 1**).

AFTERMATH OF SRI LANKAN DISASTER

Although the impact and mental health consequences of major disasters have many similarities, the nature, type, and severity can cause differences. It is helpful to conceptualize the impact along a time course of rescue, relief, rehabilitation, reconstruction, and development phases (**Table 2**). Different organizations, government departments, and international bodies like international NGOs and the UN have been responsible for the implementation of different interventions depending on the phase of the disaster. However, unlike the one-off natural tsunami, a chronic war situation did not lend itself to temporal divisions into neat phases, but was more of a continuing, complex (political) emergency going on for years with overlapping, periodic acute disaster situations for a community, like an episode of intense fighting for control of a region, a bombing raid, ambush, or a skirmish on a background of long-term displacement and then a prolonged postwar context.

Tsunami

In the immediate aftermath of the tsunami, survivors were overwhelmed, in shock, with an acute feeling of having lost everything. Acute stress reactions (ASRs) were common. ASRs typically lasted a few days. People were seen to be in a daze and highly emotional. Grief was the predominant psychological symptom. Factors that complicated grief reactions included guilt of failing to save family members. Many had repeated images of immediate family members, kin, and friends being swept away, being snatched from their hands, because they were unable to hold on. Anger and hostility were directed toward nature or the gods, at family members, or at outside agencies. Despair, crying, desolation, inability to accept what had happened, disbelief, and other emotional expressions were seen.

Anguish about missing relations when no body was recovered was common. Some recovery, relief workers, and volunteers experienced severe stress reactions and ASRs in response to traumatic experiences, such as witnessing the aftermath of the tsunami or disposing of dead bodies. There was suicidal ideation as a result of losing a large proportion of close family. Alcohol abuse was seen in men who had lost their wives and were struggling to cope with young children.

Fear of the sea and nightmares were initially common, as were fears relating to the future and the return to coastal areas. Most of the affected areas were fishing communities, and fear of the sea was expressed as "She, who gave everything, also destroyed everything." An assessment of 71 children (aged 8–15 years) undertaken 3 to 4 weeks after the tsunami in Manalkadu by trained teachers showed that 40% were at risk of developing PTSD and many others showed significant symptoms.[36]

In the first few months, minor mental health conditions like depression, anxiety-related conditions including phobias, PTSD, somatoform disorders, traumatic grief reactions, alcohol abuse, and suicidal ideas and attempts were observed. They were treated with a combination of reassurance, mobilization of support networks, listening, counseling, group work, opportunity for creative expression through art, narrations,

Table 1
Predisaster and postdisaster social ecology

	Before Conflict	Conflict	After Tsunami	After Conflict
Family	Home (veedu), nuclear, extended, united, underreported Child abuse and domestic violence	Separations, deaths, fragmentation, female-headed households	Multiple deaths, injuries, women and child casualties, destruction of home and property, camp life	Female-headed families, widows, broken homes, homeless, grief, reunification, returning combatants
Community	Village (ūr), caste and hierarchical structures, networks, traditions, rituals	Fragmentation, displacement, and refugee camps	Whole villages washed out, displacement camps	Fragmentation, resettlements, demobilization
Social processes	Cohesion, communality, patriarchy, modernization, globalization	Loss of communality, repressive ecology, female empowerment	Loss of communality, massive trauma, humanitarian help, support, breakdown of barriers and hatreds, NGO culture	Repressive ecology, powerlessness, fragmentation, female empowerment
Social effects	Changing values, loosening of traditions, family system, village, cast, gender roles; nouveau riche	Collective trauma, worldwide diaspora	Collective trauma, male alcoholism, remarriages, fostering	Collective trauma, despair, helplessness, cultural bereavement
Psychosocial interventions	Psychoeducation, participation, development, empowerment, basic mental health	Psychological first aid, psychosocial interventions, conflict resolution, peace building	Psychological first aid, grief counseling, return to earlier life patterns, psychosocial interventions	Grief counseling, reestablishing traditional structures, cultural practices, rituals, psychosocial interventions, reconciliation, rehabilitation, vocational training, income generation

From Somasundaram D. Scarred Communities: Psychosocial Impact of Manmade and Natural Disasters in Sri Lanka Society. New Delhi: SAGE; 2013, in press.

Table 2
Temporal dimension of disaster

Feature	Threat	Warning	Impact	Recoil	After Trauma
			Time		
Duration	Months	Minutes to hours	Seconds to minutes	Hours	Monthly to years
Cognition	Expectation, anticipation, worry, threat, preparation	Warning messages Emergency/denial	Shock	Relief	Inventory, loss, reality sense, coping
Emotion	Fear, anxiety, insomnia	Apprehension, arousal, panic	Panic, shock, helplessness	Daze, inhibition, numbing, euphoria, emotional release	Grief, sadness, anger, hostility, despair
Behavior	Preparatory activity	Protective action, seeking safety, displacement	Self-preservation, survival, flight or fight	Hypoactivity or hyperactivity Rescue/relief	Organized reconstruction adaptation
Mental reaction	Generalized anxiety disorder	Panic	Shock	Acute stress reaction	Phobic anxiety depression Alcohol and drug abuse Antisocial personality Development disorders Suicide
Social	Family and friends support and help. Long-term plans	Rumors, herd instinct, gathering together, evacuation	Family unity, clinging, hierarchical roles	Therapeutic community, social unity, breakdown of social barriers, loss of communality, social chaos	Refugees, rehabilitation, reconstruction, recovery, restitution, resettlement, social and cultural changes

Data from Sims AC. Neurosis in society. London: Macmillan; 1983; and Kinston W, Rosser R. Disaster: effects on mental and physical state. J Psychosom Res 1974;18:437–56.

drama, play (in children) and music, encouragement to return to habitual routines and social activities, medication when necessary, and follow-up. Individuals were observed to be more expressive of their losses, wanting to talk about them and showing signs of distress. These basic psychosocial interventions helped them recover in time. Most did not show overt mental health disorders but continued to have sleep disturbances, nightmares, and a sense of loss for varying periods of a few months.

There was an increase in relapse of schizophrenia, exacerbation of symptoms, and failure to follow regular treatment routines.[37] Some patients lost their medical records and medications in the tsunami, whereas others could not keep their clinic appointments and treatments in the posttsunami chaos. Thus, as a result of lack of regular maintenance medication and follow-up, patients with schizophrenia had relapses or deterioration in their mental condition. Some cases of schizophrenic illness or other psychotic episodes were not identified, or misidentified as reactions to the disaster, and managed inappropriately with psychological methods.

Some aspects of the systems put in place after the tsunami to deliver aid seemed to lead to more difficulties for the affected people. There was a complex official registration process to receive aid, which many found stressful. Initially, agencies were poorly organized and coordinated, and there were some cases of political interference in the supply of aid and provision of psychosocial support. Many believed that this situation led to aid and psychosocial interventions not reaching all those in need, which caused resentment and anger amongst the affected people. Initially, only a few structured activities were available in the welfare centers, and this particularly affected children and adolescents who had lost parents. As time went on, there were reports of a lack of sensitivity and sympathy in some authorities dealing with tsunami survivors, including school principals and government officials, who expected survivors to return prematurely to normal functioning.

Previous experiences of being displaced (because of conflict) and dealing with trauma seem to have prepared those affected and the relief workers to deal with the effects of the tsunami. Local traditional healers and religious communities already had experience of helping people who had suffered traumatic experiences. The combined effects of resilience as a result of previous coping experiences with trauma, and quickly mobilized community psychosocial programs, might have prevented some from developing problems needing referral to hospital-level psychiatric services. Some workers providing psychosocial support had insufficient training, and misidentified severe mental health problems needing professional help, and rather attempted to manage them on their own. Since the tsunami, some services (particularly community-based programs) have been diverted to the tsunami-affected areas, and away from areas that have a high level of psychosocial need as a result of other factors, including poverty and conflict.

War in Sri Lanka

Individuals, families, and communities in Sri Lanka, particularly in the north, the east, and the so-called border areas of Sri Lanka, have undergone 25 years of war trauma, multiple displacements, injury, detentions, torture, and loss of family, kin, friends, homes, employment, and other valued resources.[38] In addition to widespread individual mental health consequences,[39,40] such as PTSD (13%), anxiety (49%), and depression (42%) in recent internally displaced persons (IDP's) from the Vanni[39]; families and communities have been uprooted from familiar and traditional ecological contexts such as ways of life, villages, relationships, connectedness, social capital, structures, and institutions.[38] The results are termed collective trauma, which has resulted in tearing of the social fabric, lack of social cohesion, disconnection, mistrust, hopelessness, dependency, lack of motivation, powerlessness, and despondency. The social disorganization led to unpredictability, low efficacy, low social control of antisocial behavior patterns, and high emigration, which in turn cause breakdown of social norms, anomie, learned helplessness, thwarted aspirations, low self-esteem, and insecurity. Social pathologies like substance abuse, violence, gender-based abuse and child abuse have increased. Kai Erikson[41,42] gave a graphic account of collective trauma as "loss of communality" after the Buffalo Creek disaster in the United States. He and colleagues described the "broken cultures" in North American Indians and "destruction of the entire fabric of their culture" caused by the forced displacements and dispossession from traditional lands into reservations, separations, massacres, loss of their way of life, relationships, and spiritual beliefs.[43] Similar tearing of the "social fabric' has been described in Australian indigenous populations.[44]

Mental Health Services in Sri Lanka

Mental health services were not developed to meet the sudden demands of major disasters. There was insufficient recognition of disaster mental health needs or consequences. Structures or trained personnel did not exist to deal with the immense problems that were created. Our psychiatric training had not prepared us for disaster work, and knowledge of the principles of trauma and its consequences was rudimentary. Because of the massive need of patients coming for care and demand from organizations for relief of mental health problems,[45] we had to learn about disasters from the available professional literature, follow special courses, and learn from the experience of others. Because the state did not acknowledge the mental health and psychosocial consequences of war, it was left to the international and local NGOs, UN agencies, and foreign aid to fill in this gap by supporting and funding Mental Health and Psychosocial (MHPS) work.

However, after the tsunami, for the first time, the need for psychosocial work was recognized at the national level. No coordination mechanism existed, and at that time, there were no Inter-Agency Standing Committee guidelines.[46] At the local level, the preexisting and experienced primary health care and militant structures proved most effective in organizing services during the acute emergency. At the district level, spontaneous formation of committees to coordinate the psychosocial efforts (eg, the Mangrove[47] in the east, Center for Health Care in the Vanni, and the Mental Health Task Force in Jaffna[37]) was seen. Efforts were taken to organize mental health and psychosocial relief, recovery, and rehabilitation at the national level through the Center for National Operations Psychosocial Desk (and later, Task Force to Rebuild the Nation), Ministry of Health, Sri Lanka College of Psychiatrists, WHO, Consortium for Humanitarian Agencies, and many other organizations. However, links from the national level to the periphery, particularly in the north and east, for post-tsunami activities did not develop and the responses in the north (and east) were carried out in isolation from the well-resourced and well-funded programs at the national level.

IMPLICATIONS AND LESSONS LEARNED

We learned that just as disasters affect individuals, causing nonpathological distress as well as a variety of psychiatric disorders; massive and widespread trauma and loss affect family and social processes, causing changes at the family, community, and societal levels. This broader, holistic perspective becomes paramount in collectivist cultures, which have traditionally been family and community oriented, the individual tending to become submerged in the wider concerns.[48–50]

An idea of complex mental health needs at the different levels can be understood by using the WHO definition of health:

Health is a state of complete physical, mental, (familial), social, (cultural), (spiritual) and (ecological) well-being, and not merely an absence of disease or infirmity.

(WHO)

We have included the family (which is paramount in traditional Tamil society), spirituality (which is an essential part of the Tamil culture), culture, the important dimension of mental health,[51] and ecology, which arises from Bronfenbrenner's[52] and environmental models and systems theory that emphasize an overall holistic approach to the different levels, dimensions, and systems with different temporal trajectories, influencing each other to produce an interactive, dynamic (dys)functional whole (**Table 3**). The disaster itself has an impact on these systems and their interaction, and, moreover, has a temporal trajectory of its own.[53,54] More recently, a growing consensus has been emerging on the need to look at these wider dimensions to understand the dynamics of the effects of disasters and to design effective interventions,[55–57] even for western contexts in the aftermath of 9/11 and Hurricane Katrina.[58]

Because of the widespread nature of the impact of major disasters, it may be more appropriate to use public mental health approaches to deal with affected populations. Apart from the equivocal evidence on the efficacy of individualized approaches based on medications and cognitive behavioral therapy for psychiatric conditions such as PTSD,[59] the supraindividual trauma at the family and community levels in a collectivistic society would be best addressed through a community-based approach that would reach the largest population. A comprehensive and useful conceptual model (**Fig. 3**) for psychosocial and mental health interventions is an inverted pyramid, with five overlapping and interrelated levels of interventions prepared for UN and other disaster workers by the UN and International Society for Traumatic Stress Studies.[60] At the top of the pyramid are societal interventions designed for an entire population, such as laws, public safety, public policy, programs, social justice, and a free press. Descending the pyramid, interventions target progressively smaller groups of people. The next two layers concern community-level interventions, which include public education, support for community leaders, development of social infrastructure, empowerment, cultural rituals and ceremonies, service coordination, training and education of grass root workers, and capacity building. The fourth layer is family interventions, which focus both on the individual within a family context and on strategies to promote well-being of the family as a whole. The bottom layer of the pyramid concerns interventions designed for the individual with psychological symptoms or psychiatric disorders. These interventions include psychiatric, medical, and psychological treatments, which are the most expensive and labor-intensive approaches and require highly trained professional staff. The main interventions we have used are given in **Boxes 1** and **2**.

Preventive medicine uses large-scale public health measures to protect populations and eradicate or mitigate causes. Much of the deaths and destruction caused by natural disasters can be avoided. This claim is even truer for human-caused (or technological) disasters and war. In many cases of natural disasters, poor and excluded communities were located in vulnerable areas, warnings were not issued or followed, or plans were forgotten. In the heat of battle, none of the protagonists maintained maps of where they laid landmines, as they are expected to do by international

Table 3
Dimensions of health in disasters

Dimensions of Health	Causes	Symptoms	Diagnosis	Interventions
Physical	Physical injury Infections, deficiencies, excesses	Pain, fever, disability Somatization	Physical illness, psychosomatic, somatoform disorders	Drugs treatment, physiotherapy, relaxation techniques, massage
Psychological	Shock, stress Fear: terror, loss, trauma	Tension, fear, sadness, learned helplessness	ASR, PTSD, anxiety, depression, alcohol and drug abuse	Psychological first aid, psychotherapy, counseling, relaxation techniques, cognitive behavioral therapy, testimonial therapy
Family	Death, disappearance, separation Disability, poverty	Vacuum, disharmony, negative dynamics, violence, scapegoating	Family pathology	Family therapy, marital therapy, family support, family unity Cohesion, mutual understanding, relationships
Social	Unemployment, displacement, poverty, war, repressive ecology, genocide	Conflict, suicidal ideation, anomie, alienation, withdrawal, loss of communality, substance abuse, empty rituals	Parasuicide, suicide, violence, collective trauma	Group therapy, testimonio, trust Rehabilitation, community mobilization, participatory methods, empowerment, social engineering, social cohesion, building social capital, collective efficacy
Cultural	Racism, colonization, majoritarianism, cultural genocide, assimilation, domination, culture shock, acculturation stress	Depression, suicide Anger, violence Helplessness, despair Demoralization, crime	Fractured communities Drugs and alcohol Suicide, cultural bereavement, domestic violence, violence	Strengthening communities Cultural traditions, practices, healing rituals, ceremonies, traditional healers, elders, narrative therapy Recognition of the culture
Spiritual	Misfortune, bad period, spirits, angry gods, evil spells, karma	Despair, demoralization, loss of belief, loss of hope	Possession, dissociation	Logotherapy, rituals, traditional healing, meditation, contemplation, mindfulness, middle way, harmony
Ecological	Disasters, pollution, climate change, loss of biodiversity, exploitation of resources, deforestation	Epidemics, malnutrition, starvation, stress, conflict, migration, loss of communality	Pandemics, disaster syndromes, ecocide	Sustainable development, conservation, renewable energy, environmental protection, holistic and integrative methods, equilibrium, homeostasis

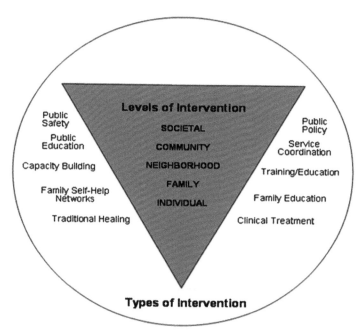

Fig. 3. Conceptual model for psychosocial interventions in social and humanitarian crises.

convention, making it more difficult for demining and safe civilian resettlement. Wars and conflict can be prevented and psychosocial well-being ensured by appropriate conflict resolution mechanisms, equitable access to resources, power sharing arrangements, social justice, and respect for human and social rights.[61] Techniques such as torture and disappearances cause long-term sequelae in individuals, their

---

Box 1
Therapeutic interventions for disaster survivors

1. Psychoeducation

2. Psychological first aid, crisis intervention

3. Psychotherapy

4. Behavioral-cognitive methods

5. Relaxation techniques

6. Pharmacotherapy

7. Group therapy

8. Family therapy

9. Expressive methods

10. Rehabilitation

11. Community approaches (see **Box 2**)

From Somasundaram D. Treatment of massive trauma due to war. Adv Psychiatr Treat 1997;3:321–31.

Box 2
Community approaches

- Psychoeducation: awareness
- Training of community workers
- Public mental health promotive activities
- Encourage indigenous coping strategies
- Cultural rituals and ceremonies
- Community interventions
  - Family
  - Groups
  - Expressive methods
  - Rehabilitation
- Prevention

---

family, and communities,[62,63] which can be prevented if international conventions, humanitarian law, and treaties are observed.

It is worthwhile planning beforehand to prevent or mitigate the impact of disasters at the community and family levels. There should be regional and international mechanisms to protect civilians in times of conflict or when powerful leaders and states overstep boundaries of good governance and observation of basic rights. Increasing powers to the UN Security Council and General Assembly to intervene with sanctions and peace-keeping forces, International Conventions and Court and the principles of right to protect[64,65] are promising developments. In the long-term, there is a need to create a culture of peace by social peace building.[66]

REFERENCES

1. Ivan V. An unfinished struggle: an investigative exposure of Sri Lanka's judiciary and the chief justice. Colombo (Sri Lanka): Ravaya; 2003.
2. University Teachers for Human Rights-Jaffna (UTHR-J). The second fascist front in Sri Lanka–towards crushing the minorities and disenfranchising the Sinhalese. In: Special reports, vol. 29. Colombo (Sri Lanka): UTHR-J; 2006. Available at: http://www.uthr.org/SpecialReports/spreport29.htm. Accessed June 22, 2013.
3. Ivan V. The harvest of 60 years of independence. Montage 2008;2:14–5.
4. Transparency International. Annual report(s). Berlin: Transparency International; 2001; 2007. Available at: http://www.transparency.org. Accessed June 22, 2013.
5. Tambiah SJ. Ethnic fratricide and the dismantling of democracy. Chicago: University of Chicago Press; 1986.
6. Cooke MC. The Lionel Bopage story–rebellion, repression and the struggle for justice in Sri Lanka. Colombo (Sri Lanka): Agahas; 2011.
7. Cordell K, Wolff S. Ethnic conflict. Cambridge (United Kingdom): Polity; 2010.
8. Marshall M, Cole B. Global report on conflict, governance and state fragility 2008. Foreign Policy Bulletin, Winter 2008;3–21.
9. Smith A. Nationalism and modernism: a critical survey of recent theories of nations and nationalism. London: Routledge; 1998.
10. Horowitz D. Ethnic groups in conflict. 2nd edition. Berkeley (CA): University of California; 2000.

11. Ross MH. Cultural contestation in ethnic conflict. Cambridge (United Kingdom): Cambridge University Press; 2007.
12. Jesse N, Williams K. Ethnic conflict–a systematic approach to cases of conflict. Washington, DC: CQ Press; 2011.
13. Esman M. An introduction to ethnic conflict. Cambridge (United Kingdom): Polity; 2004.
14. Byman D. Keeping the peace: lasting solutions to ethnic conflicts. Baltimore (MD): John Hopkins University Press; 2002.
15. Eller JD. From culture to ethnicity to conflict: an anthropological perspective on international ethnic conflict. Ann Arbor (MI): University of Michigan Press; 1999.
16. Council NP. MARGA: cost of the war. Colombo (Sri Lanka): National Peace Council; 2001.
17. Chandra K. Ethnic parties and democratic stability. Perspect Polit 2005;3: 235–52.
18. Stewart F. Horizontal inequalities: a neglected dimension of development. Oxford (United Kingdom): Centre for Research on Inequality, Human Security and Ethnicity, University of Oxford; 2001.
19. Nordstrom C. Shadows of war–violence, power, and international profiteering in the twenty-first century. Berkeley (CA): University of California Press; 2004.
20. Somasundaram D. Parallel governments–living between terror and counter terror in Northern Lanka (1982-2009). J Asian Afr Stud 2010;45:568–83.
21. Hoole M, Somasundaram D, Thiranagama R, et al. Broken palmyrah. Claremont (CA): Sri Lanka Studies Institute; 1990.
22. United Nations. Report of the Secretary-General's Internal Review Panel of the United Nations action in Sri Lanka. New York: UN; 2012. Available at: http://www.un.org/News/dh/infocus/Sri_Lanka/The_Internal_Review_Panel_report_on_Sri_Lanka.pdf. Accessed June 22, 2013.
23. University Teachers for Human Rights- Jaffna (UTHR-J). Let them speak: truth about Sri Lanka's victims of war. In: University Teachers for Human Rights-Jaffna (UTHR-J), editor. Special report. Colombo (Sri Lanka): UTHR-J; 2009. Available at: http://www.uthr.org/SpecialReports/Special%20rep34/Uthr-sp.rp34.htm. Accessed June 22, 2013.
24. Stein G. War stories. In: Segus G, editor. Dateline. Crows Nest, New South Wales (Australia): SBS; 2010. Available at: http://www.sbs.com.au/dateline/story/watch/id/600331/n/War-Stories. Accessed June 22, 2013.
25. Philp C. The hidden massacre: Sri Lanka's final offensive against Tamil Tigers. In: Times online. London: The Times; 2009. Available at: http://www.timesonline.co.uk/tol/news/world/asia/article6383449.ece. Accessed May 29, 2009.
26. Wax E. Fresh reports, imagery contradict Sri Lanka on civilian no-fire zone. In: Washington Post. Washington, DC: Washington Post; 2009. Available at: http://www.washingtonpost.com/wp-dyn/content/article/2009/05/29/AR2009052903409.html?nav=emailpage. Retrieved May 30, 2009.
27. Commission of Inquiry. Report of the commission of inquiry on lessons learnt and reconciliation. Colombo (Sri Lanka): Government of Sri Lanka; 2011. Available at: http://www.priu.gov.lk/news_update/Current_Affairs/ca201112/FINAL%20LLRC%20REPORT.pdf. Accessed June 22, 2013.
28. United Nations Secretary-General's Panel of Experts. Accountability in Sri Lanka. New York: United Nations; 2011. Available at: http://www.un.org/News/dh/infocus/Sri_Lanka/POE_Report_Full.pdf. Accessed June 22, 2013.
29. World Health Organization. Tsunami affected areas. WHO; 2005. Available at: http://www.whosrilanka.org/en/section15.htm. Accessed June 22, 2013. And

Asian Development Bank Institute (ADBI). Economic challenges of post-tsunami reconstruction in Sri Lanka. Tokyo: ABDI; 2007. Available at: http://www.adbi.org/discussion-paper/2007/08/31/2354.sri.lanka.post.tsunami.reconstruction/. Accessed June 22, 2013.

30. Frerks GK, Klem B. Tsunami response in Sri Lanka–report on a field visit from 6-20 February 2005. Wageningen (The Netherlands): Disaster Studies, Conflict Research Unit, Clingendael Institute, Wageningen University; 2005.

31. Saracento B, Minas H. Mental Health Situation in Aceh. World Health Organisation; 2005. Available at: http://www.who.int/entity/mental_health/resources/Summary_Indonesia_Strategic_plan_revised_27_Jan.pdf.

32. Galapatti A. Psychosocial work in the aftermath of the tsunami: challenges for service provision in Batticaloa, Eastern Sri Lanka. Intervention 2005;3: 65–9.

33. Wickramage K. Sri Lanka's post-tsunami psychosocial playground: lessons for future psychosocial programming and interventions following disasters. Intervention 2006;4:167–72.

34. Grewal MK. Approaches to equity in post tsunami assistance; Sri Lanka, a case study (Commissioned by the Office of the UN Special Envoy for Tsunami Recovery (OSE). London: Department for International Development, the Government of the United Kingdom; 2006. Available at: http://www.alnap.org/pool/files/ApproachestoEquity.pdf. Accessed June 22, 2013.

35. Goodhand J, Klem B, Fonseka D, et al. Aid, conflict, and peacebuilding in Sri Lanka 2000-2005. Colombo (Sri Lanka): The Asia Foundation; 2005.

36. Neuner F, Schauer E, Catani C, et al. Post-tsunami stress: a study of posttraumatic stress disorder in children living in three severely affected regions in Sri Lanka. J Trauma Stress 2006;19:339–47.

37. Danvers K, Sivayokan S, Somasundaram DJ, et al. Ten months on: qualitative assessment of psychosocial issues in Northern Sri Lanka following the tsunami. Int Psychiatr 2006;3:5–8.

38. Somasundaram D. Collective trauma in Northern Sri Lanka: a qualitative psychosocial-ecological study. Int J Ment Health Syst 2007;1:5.

39. Husain F, Anderson M, Cardozo BL, et al. Prevalence of war-related mental health conditions and association with displacement status in postwar Jaffna District, Sri Lanka. JAMA 2011;306:522–31.

40. Somasundaram D, Sivayokan S. War trauma in a civilian population. Br J Psychiatry 1994;165:524–7.

41. Erikson K. Disaster at Buffalo Creek. Loss of communality at Buffalo Creek. Am J Psychiatry 1976;133:302–5.

42. Erikson K. In the wake of the flood. London: Allen Unwin; 1979.

43. Erikson K, Vecsey C. A report to the people of grassy narrows. In: Vecsey C, Venables R, editors. American Indian environments– ecological issues in Native American history. New York: Syracuse University Press; 1980. p. 152–61.

44. Milroy H. Australian Indigenous Doctors' Association (AIDA) submissions on the consultative document: preventative healthcare and strengthening Australia's social and economic fabric. Submission to National Health and Medical Research Council (NHMRC), Australia. 2005.

45. Somasundaram D. Scarred minds. New Delhi (India): Sage; 1998.

46. Inter-Agency Standing Committee (IASC). IASC Guidelines on mental health and psychosocial support in emergency settings. Geneva (Switzerland): WHO; 2007. Available at: http://www.who.int/mental_health/emergencies/guidelines_iasc_mental_health_psychosocial_june_2007.pdf. Accessed June 22, 2013.

47. Mangrove. The Mangrove: psychosocial support and coordination network, Batticaloa. Batticaloa (Sri Lanka): Mangrove; 2006. Available at: http://www.themangrove.blogspot.com/. Accessed June 22, 2013.

48. Yeh C, Arora A, Wu K. A new theoretical model of collectivistic coping. In: Wong P, Wong L, editors. Handbook of multicultural perspectives on stress and coping. New York: Springer; 2006. p. 56–72.

49. De Jong J. Public mental health and culture: disasters as a challenge to western mental health care models, the self, and PTSD. In: Wilson J, Drozdek B, editors. Broken spirits: the treatment of asylum seekers and refugees with PTSD. New York: Brunner/Routledge; 2004. p. 159–79.

50. Hofstede G. Cultures and organizations: software of the mind. 2nd edition. New York: McGraw-Hill; 2005. 2008.

51. Bhugra D, Bhui K, editors. Textbook of cultural psychiatry. Cambridge (United Kingdom): Cambridge University Press; 2007. p. 561–7.

52. Bronfenbrenner U. The ecology of human development: experiments by nature and design. Cambridge (MA): Harvard University Press; 1979.

53. Sims AC. Neurosis in society. London: Macmillan; 1983.

54. Kinston W, Rosser R. Disaster: effects on mental and physical state. J Psychosom Res 1974;18:437–56.

55. Landau J, Saul J. Facilitating family and community resilience in response to major disaster. In: Walsh F, McGoldrick M, editors. Living beyond loss. New York: Norton; 2004. p. 285–309.

56. De Jong J. Public mental health, traumatic stress and human rights violations in low-income countries: a culturally appropriate model in times of conflict, disaster and peace. In: De Jong J, editor. Trauma, war and violence: public mental health in sociocultural context. New York: Plenum-Kluwer; 2002. p. 1–91.

57. Psychosocial Working Group. Psychosocial intervention in complex emergencies: a conceptual framework (University of Edinburgh ed). Edinburgh (United Kingdom): Psychosocial Working Group; 2003.

58. Saul J, Bava S. Implementing collective approaches to massive trauma/loss in western contexts: implications for recovery, peacebuilding and development. In: Hamber B, editor. Trauma, development, and peacebuilding: towards an integrated psychosocial approach. New Delhi (India): International Conflict Research Institute, in press.

59. Institute of Medicine (IOM). Treatment of posttraumatic stress disorder: an assessment of the evidence. Washington, DC: National Academies of Sciences; 2008. Available at: http://www.nap.edu/catalog/11955.html. Accessed June 22, 2013.

60. Green B, Friedman M, de Jong J, editors. Trauma, interventions in war and peace: prevention, practice, and policy. New York: Kluwer/Plenum Press; 2003.

61. Psychosocial Assessment of Development and Humanitarian Interventions (PADHI). A tool, a guide, and a framework. Colombo (Sri Lanka): PADHI; 2009.

62. Doney A. The psychological after-effects of torture: a survey of Sri Lankan ex. detainees. In: Somasundaram D, editor. Scarred minds. New Delhi (India): Sage; 1998. p. 256–87.

63. Somasundaram D. Psycho-social aspects of torture in Sri Lanka. Int J Cult Ment Health 2008;1:10–23.

64. Evans G. The limits of state sovereignty: the responsibility to protect in the 21st century. In: Eighth Neelam Tiruchelvam memorial lecture by Gareth Evans, president, International Crisis Group. Colombo (Sri Lanka): International

Centre for Ethnic Studies (ICES); 2007. Available at: http://www.crisisgroup.org/en/publication-type/speeches/2007/evans-the-limits-of-state-sovereignty-the-responsibility-to-protect-in-the-21st-century.aspx. Accessed June 22, 2013.

65. Evans G. The responsibility to protect–ending mass atrocity crises once and for all. Washington, DC: Brookings Institution Press; 2008.

66. Large J. Considering conflict. In: First health as a bridge for peace consultative meeting; 30–31 October 1997. Les Pensières, Annecy: WHO; 1997.

The Psychological and Psychiatric Effects of Terrorism
Lessons from London

G. James Rubin, PGCAP, MSc, PhD*,
Simon Wessely, MA, BM, BCh, MSc, MD, FRCP, FRCPsych, FMedSci, FKC

KEYWORDS

- Psychological effects • Psychiatric effects • Bombing • Terrorism

KEY POINTS

- Distress in the community is common, but is likely to fade with time and does not usually require clinical intervention.
- Providing information and facilitating communication between people can reduce levels of distress in the community.
- Most people who develop a psychiatric disorder following a disaster do not find their way into treatment via the usual referral routes.
- Targeted outreach efforts are effective in finding people who have developed a psychiatric disorder and in helping them access appropriate, evidence-based treatment.

BACKGROUND

As with many major European cities, London has witnessed its share of war and terrorism within living memory. In particular, nearly 30,000 Londoners died between 1940 and 1941 during the Blitz. Although Government officials at the time were deeply concerned about the potentially devastating effect a bombing campaign might have on public morale, in practice little evidence was found of the expected panic among the general public, and commentators were surprised to note that "one of the most striking things about the effects of the war on the civilian population has been the relative rarity of pathological mental disturbances among the civilians exposed to air-raids."[1,2] Although debate continues about the true short-term social effects of the Blitz on the London population, the concept of a Blitz spirit,

Funding: None.
Conflicts of Interest: None.
King's College London, Department of Psychological Medicine, Weston Education Centre, Cutcombe Road, London SE5 9RJ, UK
* Corresponding author.
E-mail address: gideon.rubin@kcl.ac.uk

Psychiatr Clin N Am 36 (2013) 339–350
http://dx.doi.org/10.1016/j.psc.2013.05.008
0193-953X/13/$ – see front matter © 2013 Elsevier Inc. All rights reserved.

psych.theclinics.com

encapsulating notions of stoicism and solidarity, remains a strong cultural reference point within Britain and one that is regularly called on by commentators and politicians during times of crisis.

From the 1960s to the late 1990s, the so-called Troubles in Northern Ireland brought bombs back to the streets of London. The Troubles resulted in more than 3500 deaths as a result of actions by Republican and Loyalist paramilitary groups and official security forces.[3] Although most deaths occurred in Northern Ireland, many high-profile attacks also occurred in cities within the United Kingdom, including London, until the Good Friday agreement of 1998 committed all the main groups to putting violence behind them.

However, as memories of the Irish Republican Army started to fade, a new threat began to encroach on public consciousness: that from Al Qaeda and Islamic extremism. The events of 11 September 2001 meant that the skies of London were also empty for a week, and once the UK Armed Forces were committed to participating in the invasion of Iraq in the spring of 2003, threat assessments increased and senior politicians and security officials repeatedly warned the public that an attack from this new threat was highly likely, if not inevitable. In August 2004 a leaflet was sent to every home in the country with advice on what to do in the event of a major incident. These warnings proved accurate. On 6 July 2005, news that London had been awarded the 2012 Summer Olympic and Paralympic Games brought crowds to Trafalgar Square to celebrate. The next day, terrorists loosely linked to Al Qaeda detonated 4 suicide bombs on the London transport system.

THE EVENTS OF JULY 2005

The 4 bombers detonated their bombs during the morning rush hour (**Fig. 1**). Three bombs exploded almost simultaneously, at 08:50, on 3 different crowded underground trains. The fourth exploded an hour later, in Tavistock Square, on one of London's iconic double-decker buses. Tavistock Square had been the London home of the writer Virginia Woolf, who recorded in her diaries returning to the Square after a night of bombing in October 1940 to find her own home devastated. The 2005 bombs killed 56 people (including the four bombers) and injured 784.[4] Despite initial confusion as to the cause of the explosions, news of the attacks was quickly disseminated to the wider public, who were initially asked to remain where they were and not to travel within central London until further notice. This all-clear was provided by midafternoon, although public transport remained heavily disrupted.

Over the weeks that followed, a substantial and highly visible police presence was deployed within London. Despite this, 2 weeks later, on 21 July, an apparently separate Al Qaeda–inspired terrorist cell attempted to use 4 more bombs on the London transport system: 3 on underground trains and 1 on a bus. This time, although the detonator caps went off, the main explosives failed and no one was injured. As part of the subsequent manhunt, on the next day police misidentified an innocent man, Jean Charles de Menezes, as one of the suspected terrorists and shot him dead after he boarded an underground train. Over the subsequent month, the real would-be bombers, together with several others, were found and arrested. They are currently serving life sentences.

THE ACUTE PSYCHOLOGICAL IMPACT

Evidence on how Londoners in general reacted to the events of July 2005 comes largely from 2 telephone surveys commissioned by our team. The first used conventional market research techniques to collect data from 1010 randomly selected adult

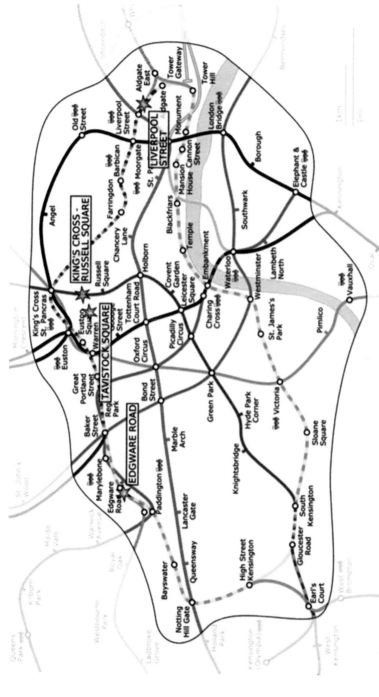

Fig. 1. London map with bombing sites indicated. (*Courtesy of British Red Cross, London, United Kingdom.*)

members of the London population.[5] Interviews took place between 18 and 20 July. Proportional quota sampling, with quotas based on sex, age, working status, residential location, housing tenure, and ethnicity, were used to ensure that the eventual sample was demographically representative of the population of London. Eight-hundred and fifteen of these participants gave us permission to speak to them again and 7 to 8 months later (between 3 February and 5 March 2006) we reinterviewed 574 of them.[6]

Our primary outcome for this research was a measure composed of 5 stress-related symptoms that was initially used to assess reactions among the US population to the 11 September 2001 attacks.[7] These symptoms were:

1. Feeling upset when reminded of the 7 July bombings
2. Repeated disturbing memories, thoughts, or dreams about it
3. Having difficulty concentrating
4. Trouble falling or staying asleep
5. Feeling irritable or having angry outbursts

Participants were asked whether they had experienced each of these not at all, a little bit, moderately, quite a bit, or extremely as a result of the London bombings. The interpretation of high scores on this measure as indicating a clinically relevant level of distress that warrants treatment has been criticized, not least by us.[8] However, as a measure of upset or distress, such scales are useful in providing a guide to the psychological state of the public and for identifying factors that reduce or exacerbate psychological responses to a major incident.[9]

In our first survey, 2 weeks after the attacks, 31% of respondents reported experiencing one or more stress-related symptoms quite a bit or extremely. In comparison, 44% of participants in the US survey responded in this way in the immediate aftermath of the 11 September attacks.[7] Perceptions of safety were also affected by the attack: 55% of our respondents thought that their lives were currently in danger from terrorism; 86% thought (correctly, as it turned out) that another attack on London was likely in the near future; 46% thought they were unsafe when traveling by Underground; and 33% thought they were unsafe when going into central London. Linked to this reduced sense of safety, intended avoidance of public transport and of central London was also high: 30% of Underground users reported that they would now use the Underground less once the transport system returned to normal, whereas 20% reported that they now intended to visit central London less often. Entrance data from London Underground stations have subsequently been analyzed and suggest that these intentions translated into avoidance behavior.[10]

Although these figures suggest that the attacks caused a clear psychological shock to London, the decline in stress-related symptoms in the US population following 11 September 2001[11] led us to expect a similar decline in the months following the 7 July bombings. Our follow-up data confirmed this. Seven months after the attacks, only 11% of respondents reported experiencing one or more psychological symptoms quite a bit or extremely as a result of the bombings. Despite this, it was notable that many people still thought that they were under threat: 52% thought that their own lives were in danger from terrorism, whereas 90% thought that another attack was likely in the near future.

As is common in surveys of risk perception, participants' perceptions of the risk from terrorism tended to be higher for their loved ones than for themselves. Linked to this, a strong desire existed on the day of the attacks for people to make contact with their friends and family to reassure themselves that they were well; again, this is a well-recognized finding from disaster research.[12] However, the demand that this placed on the mobile phone networks made communication difficult and 78% of our participants who tried contacting others on the day reported finding it difficult to get through. This difficulty had psychological implications, with those who found it difficult to make contact with others on their mobile phones being significantly more likely to report symptoms of distress.

Problems with communication between people also had implications for the emergency services. When people were unable to find out whether their loved ones were safe, many attempted to contact the police Casualty Bureau telephone line in an attempt to locate them. At its peak, the Bureau received 43,000 attempted phone calls per hour, more than could be handled.[13] As well as handling calls about missing people, the Bureau also fielded enquiries about a range of other issues, including public transport arrangements. Many worried relatives and friends of missing people who were unable to get through to the Bureau or to obtain information then attempted to call or visit hospitals in an attempt to find out more.[13] These efforts added an unnecessary burden to hospital staff who were already under intense pressure and were therefore often unable to provide suitable advice or support to anxious relatives. Similar surges of family members and low-risk patients toward health care facilities have previously been observed in several different contexts and often prove problematic.[14–17]

The desire to contact family members and ensure their safety also extended to parents. Despite widely disseminated police advice that members of the public should not travel in central London until the all-clear was given, 26% of parents in our survey who had a child in school on that day reported going to school earlier than usual to collect or see their children. Although this had no health implications during the London bombings, had the attack involved a chemical, biological, or radiological component, this response might have increased the exposure of the parents and children to danger. Recent focus groups by our team suggest that a similar lack of compliance with police advice by parents is likely following a so-called dirty bomb attack unless improved communication about the safety of children at school is provided.[18]

As well as trying to reassure themselves about the safety of others, in the weeks following the attack people used their social support networks to discuss their emotional responses, with 71% of participants saying that they had talked with someone else about their thoughts and feelings about what happened. In contrast, less than 1% reported speaking to a mental health professional. Given that early mental health interventions to prevent the development of posttraumatic stress disorder are at best ineffective and at worst detrimental,[19] we were reassured by this finding.

Our survey also found some intriguing evidence that London's prior history with terrorism provided the population with some protection against the emotional effects of the 7 July attacks, with the 30% of respondents who had previously been caught up in a terrorist incident or a false alarm about terrorism being less likely to experience distress. The Government's earlier attempt to improve resilience by providing households with information about what to do in a major incident was less effective. Despite being sent to every household in the country less than a year earlier, only 37% of our respondents could recall having read it. Moreover, reading the leaflet did not reduce the likelihood of experiencing distress immediately following the attacks and neither was it associated with having made the specific practical preparations for a disaster that were recommended in the leaflet.[20]

In the short term, the strongest predictors of distress were demographic and exposure related. Distress was most common among participants from ethnic minority groups: Muslims (compared with other religious groups), poorer participants, those who thought that they might have been injured or killed, and those for whom a close friend or relative had been injured or killed. These results are largely in line with other research showing that disadvantaged groups and those with higher levels of exposure tend to experience greater psychological and psychiatric effects after a disaster,[21] although the association between being Muslim and experiencing higher levels of distress may be a specific feature of this form of Al Qaeda–inspired terrorism. Although it is only possible to speculate as to the reasons for the association involving Muslims, it is plausible that fears of a backlash against Muslim communities were important. In terms of psychological state as measured in our follow-up survey, only being poorer and having feared that a family member or friend might have been injured or killed predicted whether a participant still experienced distress 7 months later.

Although our surveys provided good evidence about reactions among the general community, evidence concerning the acute psychological impact of the attacks on those more directly exposed to them is limited. In an analysis of newspaper accounts, eyewitness testimony, and interviews with witnesses and survivors, Drury and colleagues[22] identified little, if any, evidence of panic or selfish behavior among commuters on the bombed trains and bus in the initial minutes and hours following the explosions, a finding that has been observed in many other contexts.[23,24] As with other incidents, accounts instead tended to describe survivors helping each other, providing reassurance, and feeling a sense of unity with those who only moments early had been strangers.

Emotional and practical support in the subsequent days and weeks for those directly affected by the attacks was centered around a Family Assistance Centre that was set up in London to provide a gateway through which people could access emotional support and advice, assistance in making contact with other agencies, financial and legal advice, and other services (**Fig. 2**). Although the center was highly regarded by those who used it, there was some initial confusion over the remit of the center because of the misleading nature of its name. All those affected, and not just families, were welcome, resulting its subsequent renaming as the 7th July Assistance Centre. In addition, the limited budget available for promoting the center's services have left some doubts as to whether all of those who might have benefited from it were made aware of its existence.[25] In our survey, few people recognized it.

However, a note of caution is appropriate at this point regarding the reliability of surveys of public awareness of postdisaster services. In our survey we not only asked respondents whether they were aware of the 7th July Assistance Centre but also whether they were aware of the NHS Trauma Response Program (discussed later),

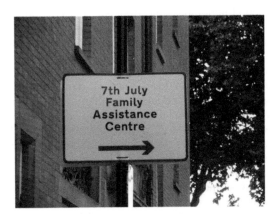

Fig. 2. Family Assistance Centre sign.

NHS (National Health Service) Direct, and the London Rescue Program. The London Rescue Program had the highest recognition, with 37% of respondents indicating that they were aware of it. However, it was also the one that was fictitious.

POSTACUTE PSYCHIATRIC IMPACT AND RESPONSE

Although the psychological impact of July 2005 eventually faded for most members of the public, as with any disaster or terrorist attack a minority were left with longer-term symptoms that disrupted their quality of life. Following previous terrorist attacks, it has been apparent that most people who might benefit from treatment of their mental health problems do not actively seek care.[26] In order to meet the potentially large unmet public mental health need following the 7 July bombings, a novel 2-year strategy was funded by the Department of Health to screen those people who had been directly exposed to potentially traumatic events and to offer evidence-based treatments to those found to have a psychiatric disorder. Full details and evaluation of this Trauma Response Program have been provided elsewhere.[27–29]

In brief, a central screening and assessment team, staffed by a psychiatrist, 2 psychological assistants, and an administrator, used a variety of methods to make contact with as many as possible of the estimated 4000 people who had been directly caught up in the attacks. Lists of those affected were obtained from hospitals that had treated victims, charities providing support to victims, the Health Protection Agency, and via a dedicated telephone support line. In addition, the service was advertised to people attending the 7th July Assistance Centre, via police witness lists and through a mass-media campaign. All general practitioners within London were sent 2 letters informing and reminding them of the existence of the service. Everyone identified in this way was asked to complete a short questionnaire that contained 10 questions about the presence of symptoms associated with posttraumatic stress disorder (the Trauma Screening Questionnaire[30]), 2 questions about symptoms of depression, 3 questions about travel phobia and increased smoking or alcohol consumption, and 1 question about any other response to the bombings that the person was concerned about. Those who screened positive to the Trauma Screening Questionnaire or any other items were invited for a more detailed clinical assessment and were either referred on for immediate treatment or were asked to complete additional screening questionnaires after 3, 6, and 9 months. By the end of the screening period, 910 people were contacted by the team. These people were almost entirely identified through the active acquisition of lists from other agencies. Only 5.8% of people self-referred, 3.3% were referred by friends or relatives, and 4.3% were referred by general practitioners. Had the team not engaged in active outreach efforts, it is probable that most of those eventually treated by the program would have remained unknown to mental health services. Five-hundred and ninety-six people returned a screening questionnaire, of whom 56.7% screened positive. In total, 248 people were eventually referred for treatment to the 3 clinical teams taking part in the Trauma Response Program. Two-hundred and seventeen entered treatment, and 189 completed treatment. Posttraumatic stress disorder was the most common primary diagnosis in patients, although travel phobia, depression, adjustment disorder, complicated grief, and generalized anxiety disorder were also observed.[28]

Treatments used for patients with posttraumatic stress disorder were trauma-focused cognitive behavior therapy (for more than 80% of patients), eye movement desensitization and reprocessing (10%), and a combination of both therapies (10%). Other disorders were treated with the most appropriate evidence-based therapy, mainly cognitive behavior therapy. All patients completed validated measures of posttraumatic and depression symptoms before and during treatment. A smaller subset also completed follow-up measures. Subsequent analyses of these data suggested that the improvements in mental health that were observed in treated patients were equivalent to the effect sizes observed in randomized controlled trials of multi-session cognitive behavior therapy for adults with posttraumatic stress disorder.[28] The treatments offered by the program therefore worked.

The proactive screen-and-treat approach adopted by the Trauma Response Program was an innovative and largely successful public mental health response to the 7 July bombings. However, because it was novel and had to be put in place quickly following the attack, there are aspects of it that could be improved on in any future response. Three opportunities for refinement are worth particular attention.

First, the process of assembling a list of people who had been directly involved in the attacks and who were most at risk of developing a psychiatric illness was unnecessarily complicated. No single official agency took responsibility for assembling such a list, and sharing of information between agencies was hampered by an overly cautious interpretation of legislation designed to safeguard personal data.[13] As a result, the Trauma Response Program was only able to contact 910 out of the estimated 4000 people exposed to the attacks. Within the United Kingdom, greater clarity about the flexibility that emergency responders have under existing legislation to share information with others has now been provided,[31] and the Health Protection Agency has been given responsibility for setting up a registry of those affected by a future attack or disaster, to facilitate health screening. One of the 11 factors suggested as a suitable rationale for setting up such a register is that "there is a reasonable possibility of short or long-term physical and/or psychological health effects among the exposed population."[32]

Second, issues around the sensitivity of the screening questionnaire have been raised.[29] Although the questionnaire had been found to work well in other contexts, the high levels of stress in the general community after the 7 July attacks reduced its specificity during the early stages of the Trauma Response Program. The higher levels of stress in people from ethnic minority groups also meant that a larger proportion of people who did not have a psychiatric disorder were identified as possible cases among these groups than amongst the white majority group.[29] Although genuine cases continued to be identified accurately in all subgroups over the lifetime of the program, the reduced efficiency in the early stages and among survivors from ethnic minorities meant that additional resources had to be spent assessing people who did not require treatment.

Third, although the use of both cognitive behavior therapy and eye movement desensitization and reprocessing was justified based on the best available evidence, it could be argued that an opportunity was lost to compare the relative merits of these two approaches. The Trauma Response team noted that the ethical, financial, and organizational constraints involved in putting together a clinical trial during an unplanned response to a crisis, together with a desire to overcome barriers to treatment, prevented them from running a randomized controlled trial comparing the two treatments,[28] and this is a fair justification. Looking to the future, if such a program is to be repeated in the United Kingdom or elsewhere following the next disaster or terrorist attack, there is no reason in principle why arrangements could not be made in advance to set up randomized controlled trials that can be integrated in future responses. These trials do not necessarily need to be restricted to evaluation of treatments. For example, integrated studies to evaluate different approaches to encouraging the return of screening questionnaires would be equally informative and need not present substantial ethical or organizational dilemmas.

IMPLICATIONS FOR FUTURE DISASTER MENTAL HEALTH RESPONSES

Several organizations have tried to identify lessons from London's experiences with the events of July 2005.[13,25,31,33] Our suggestions for what might be learned regarding disaster mental health responses are as follows:

1. Following any disaster, addressing the basic needs of the affected community is an important way of reducing distress. The need for information should not be overlooked. In mass casualty incidents, members of the public have a pressing need to reassure themselves that their loved ones are safe. If this is not possible, levels of distress increase and emergency services may need to divert attention from dealing with casualties to providing advice and information to worried relatives who are seeking information. Providing resilient mobile telecommunications infrastructure, ensuring that members of the public know to keep mobile phone calls brief to free up capacity for others, and encouraging people to use social media where possible should help to minimize this effect.

2. Other, more basic, information needs also need to be addressed. Depending on the incident, people may have questions such as what region is affected, what transport options are available, what the public are being advised to do, how children at school are being kept safe, and so on. Again, if such needs are not explicitly tackled, emergency services may have to divert resources to provide this basic level of advice at an individual level or deal with changes in public behavior that run contrary to official advice. Uncertainty about the facts of an incident is also likely to lead to higher levels of distress, particular if a chemical, biological, or radiological component is suspected.[34,35] The questions people will have, and the types of answers they will find acceptable, can and should be predicted in advance.[36] Ensuring that information is disseminated effectively requires a stepped system of communication using multiple trusted spokespeople. This strategy should use the mass media; social media; community networks; automated telephone help lines; and, for those who still require more information, manned telephone help lines to divert members of the public away from seeking information in person at health care facilities. Advertising these information sources is as important as providing them.[37,38]

3. Although distress and behavior change in the general community is to be expected, most people access their own preexisting social support networks to talk about their experiences. Psychological changes fade over time for most people. It remains difficult to predict with any accuracy who will develop a longer-term psychiatric disorder. Nonetheless, it is possible to identify specific sections of society in which the psychological effects of a disaster will be strongest and to target communication and support accordingly. In particular, the concerns of groups that are likely to be stigmatized or to face a backlash following a major incident should be considered.

4. Rapid psychosocial surveillance techniques can assist in identifying levels of distress, information needs, and awareness of services in the community. A basic structure for this type of surveillance should be developed in advance. Although it was possible to use conventional telephone surveys for this purpose following the 7 July bombings, more extreme disasters may disrupt telecommunications or displace affected populations, adding substantial complexity to this work.[39]

5. For those most affected by a disaster, a dedicated assistance center that can help with pragmatic advice and support is useful. If possible, such centers should be planned for in advance and appropriately advertised to affected people.

6. Waiting for patients who have a disaster-related psychiatric disorder to access mental health services is ineffective. Outreach efforts are required to ensure that

those who are most likely to require treatment are identified, assessed, and offered appropriate, evidence-based treatment. The screen-and-treat model adopted in London offers a good approach from which to build.

7. Screening people who are most at risk of developing a psychiatric disorder requires access to a comprehensive list of victims, witnesses, and responders. Assembling this list is therefore an essential component of the mental health response to a disaster, but requires explicit, preexisting agreements between responding agencies as to who will take responsibility for assembling it and how personal contact details will be shared with other agencies. Official agencies must not wait until after a disaster occurs to begin discussing these issues.

8. The integration of research within London's Trauma Response Program should be seen as one of its major achievements. Although providing evidence-based treatments is important, plans should also be made to assess their impacts to inform the refinement of the service and the implementation of any future disaster response. Early consideration is recommended of whether and how to incorporate experimental designs into a disaster response to answer important questions and provide better care for patients.

REFERENCES

1. Jones E, Woolven R, Durodie B, et al. Civilian morale during the Second World War: responses to air raids re-examined. Soc Hist Med 2004;17:463–79.
2. Jones E, Woolven R, Durodie B, et al. Public panic and morale: Second World War civilian responses re-examined in the light of the current anti-terrorist campaign. J Risk Res 2006;9:57–73.
3. University of Ulster. Conflict archive on the Internet. Available at: http://cain.ulst. ac.uk/index.html. Accessed December 18, 2012.
4. Anonymous. Report of the official account of the bombings in London on 7th July 2005. London: The Stationery Office; 2012.
5. Rubin GJ, Brewin CR, Greenberg N, et al. Psychological and behavioural reactions to the bombings in London on 7 July 2005: cross sectional survey of a representative sample of Londoners. BMJ 2005;331:606.
6. Rubin GJ, Brewin CR, Greenberg N, et al. Enduring consequences of terrorism: 7 month follow-up survey of reactions to the bombings in London on 7 July 2005. Br J Psychiatry 2007;190:350–6.
7. Schuster MA, Stein BD, Jaycox LH, et al. A national survey of stress reactions after the September 11, 2001, terrorist attacks. N Engl J Med 2001;345:1507–12.
8. Wessely S. When being upset is not a mental health disorder. Psychiatry 2004;67: 153–7.
9. Rubin GJ, Amlôt R, Page L, et al. Methodological challenges in assessing general population reactions in the immediate aftermath of a terrorist attack. Int J Methods Psychiatr Res 2008;17:S29–35.
10. Prager F, Beeler Asay GR, Lee B, et al. Exploring reductions in London underground passenger journeys following the July 2005 bombings. Risk Anal 2011; 31:773–86.
11. Stein BD, Elliott MN, Jajcox LH, et al. A national longitudinal study of the psychological consequences of the September 11, 2001 terrorist attacks: reactions, impairment, and help-seeking. Psychiatry 2004;67:105–17.
12. Bleich A, Gelkopf M, Solomon Z. Exposure to terrorism, stress-related mental health symptoms, and coping behaviors among a nationally representative sample in Israel. JAMA 2003;290:612–20.

13. HM Government. Addressing lessons from the emergency response to the 7 July 2005 London bombings. What we learned and what we are doing about it. Norwich (United Kingdom): Her Majesty's Stationery Office; 2006.

14. Rubin GJ, Amlôt R, Rogers MB, et al. Public perceptions of and reactions to pneumonic plague. Emerg Infect Dis 2010;16:120–2.

15. Rubin GJ, Dickmann P. How to reduce the impact of "low risk patients" following a bioterrorist incident: lessons from SARS, anthrax and pneumonic plague. Biosecur Bioterror 2010;8:37–43.

16. Pearce JM, Rubin GJ, Amlôt R, et al. Communicating public health advice following a chemical spill: results from national surveys in the UK and Poland. Disaster Med Public Health Prep 2012. http://dx.doi.org/10.1001/dmp.2012.57.

17. Rubin GJ, Potts HW, Michie S. The impact of communications about swine flu (influenza A H1N1v) on public responses to the outbreak: results from 36 national telephone surveys in the UK. Health Technol Assess 2010;14:183–266.

18. Rogers MB, Amlôt R, Rubin GJ. Investigating the impact of communication materials on public responses to a radiological dispersal device (RDD) attack. Biosecur Bioterror 2013;11:49–58.

19. Rose S, Bisson J, Wessely S. A systematic review of single-session psychological interventions ('debriefing') following trauma. Psychother Psychosom 2003;72: 176–84.

20. Page L, Rubin J, Amlôt R, et al. Are Londoners prepared for an emergency? A longitudinal study following the London bombings. Biosecur Bioterror 2008;6:309–19.

21. Whalley MG, Brewin CR. Mental health following terrorist attacks. Br J Psychiatry 2007;190:94–6.

22. Drury J, Cocking C, Reicher S. The nature of collective resilience: survivor reactions to the 2005 London bombings. Int J Mass Emerg Disasters 2009;27:66–95.

23. Sheppard B, Rubin GJ, Wardman JK, et al. Terrorism and dispelling the myth of a panic prone public. J Public Health Policy 2006;27:219–45.

24. Glass TA, Spoch-Spana M. Bioterrorism and the people: how to vaccinate a city against panic. Clin Infect Dis 2001;34:217–23.

25. Nicholls S, Healy C. Communication with disaster survivors: towards best practice. Aust J Emerg Manag 2008;23:20.

26. Stuber J, Galea S, Boscarino JA, et al. Was there unmet mental health need after the September 11, 2001 terrorist attacks? Soc Psychiatry Psychiatr Epidemiol 2006;40:1–11.

27. Brewin CR, Scragg P, Robertson M, et al. Promoting mental health following the London bombings: a screen and treat approach. J Trauma Stress 2008;2:3–8.

28. Brewin CR, Fuchkan N, Huntley Z, et al. Outreach and screening following the 2005 London bombings: usage and outcomes. Psychol Med 2010;40:2049–57.

29. Brewin CR, Fuchkan N, Huntley Z. Diagnostic accuracy of the trauma screening questionnaire after the 2005 London bombings. J Trauma Stress 2010;23:393–8.

30. Brewin CR, Rose S, Andrews B, et al. Brief screening instrument for post-traumatic stress disorder. Br J Psychiatry 2002;181:158–62.

31. HM Government. Data protection and sharing - guidance for emergency planners and responders. London: Cabinet Office; 2007.

32. Paranthaman K, Catchpole M, Simpson J, et al. Developing a decision framework for establishing a health register following a major incident. Prehospital Disaster Med 2012;27:1–7.

33. Brewin CR. Mental health response to disasters. Health Serv J 2010. Available at: http://www.hsj.co.uk/resource-centre/your-ideas-and-suggestions/mental-health-response-to-disasters/5012491.article. Accessed December 18, 2012.

34. Rubin GJ, Amlôt R, Wessely S, et al. Anxiety, distress and anger among British nationals following the Fukushima nuclear accident. Br J Psychiatry 2012;201: 400–7.

35. Rogers MB, Amlôt R, Rubin GJ, et al. Mediating the social and psychological impact of terrorist attacks: the role of risk perception and risk communication. Int Rev Psychiatry 2007;19:279–88.

36. Rubin GJ, Chowdhury A, Amlôt R. How to communicate with the public following a chemical, biological, radiological or nuclear attack: a systematic review. Biosecur Bioterror 2012;10:383–95.

37. Rubin GJ, Page LA, Morgan O, et al. Public information needs after the poisoning of Alexander Litvinenko with polonium-210 in London: cross sectional telephone survey and qualitative analysis. BMJ 2007;335:1143–6.

38. Rubin GJ, Amlôt R, Carter H, et al. Reassuring and managing patients with concerns about swine flu: qualitative interviews with callers to NHS direct. BMC Public Health 2010;10:45.

39. Kessler RC, Keane TM, Mokdad A, et al. Sample and design consideration in post-disaster mental health needs assessment tracking surveys. Int J Methods Psychiatr Res 2008;17(Suppl 2):S6–20.

The Great East Japan Earthquake, Tsunami, and Fukushima Daiichi Nuclear Power Plant Accident

A Triple Disaster Affecting the Mental Health of the Country

Jun Yamashita, PhD[a],*, Jun Shigemura, MD, PhD[b]

KEYWORDS

- The Great East Japan Earthquake • Tohoku region • Tsunami
- Fukushima Daiichi nuclear power plant accident • Psychological First Aid

KEY POINTS

- Posttraumatic stress disorder, major depressive disorder, and suicide need to be monitored closely in the wake of the Great East Japan Earthquake. Other problems include compassion fatigue among caregivers and discrimination against Fukushima residents, including workers in the nuclear power plant.
- Outreach activities of public health teams (eg, setting up common rooms) in temporary housing developments have been found effective in dealing with scarce mental health resources in the Tohoku region and in reducing psychological barriers because of stigma around receiving treatment. Japan now advocates education of first responders with Psychological First Aid.
- Future disaster response efforts in Japan should include mental health measures in the national disaster plans, and a review of subsidized or reimbursed psychotherapy for evacuees provided by professionals outside doctors' offices. Agreement about methods of training and supervising mental health professionals should be developed in Japan.

In 2011 Japan experienced one of the biggest earthquakes in the last 1000 years. The Great East Japan Earthquake was record-breaking itself and caused 2 other serious disasters: a tsunami and a nuclear power plant accident. The tsunami destroyed the past of its victims while the nuclear power plant accident threatens their future, and

Disclosure of Interests: None.
[a] Faculty of Letters, Department of Humanities and Social Sciences, Keio University, Tokyo, Japan; [b] Department of Psychiatry, National Defense Medical College, 3-2 Namiki, Tokorozawa, Saitama 359-8513, Japan
* Corresponding author. Department of Drug Informatics, Graduate School of Pharmaceutical Sciences, Chiba University, 1-8-1 InoHana, Chuo-ku, Chiba, 260-8675 Japan.
E-mail addresses: yamajun37@gmail.com; yamajun@chiba-u.jp

Psychiatr Clin N Am 36 (2013) 351–370
http://dx.doi.org/10.1016/j.psc.2013.05.004
0193-953X/13/$ – see front matter © 2013 Elsevier Inc. All rights reserved.

the earthquake continues to add stress to the present lives of survivors in the Fukushima, Iwate, and Miyagi prefectures in the Tohoku region, located 200 to 500 km (125–310 miles) northeast of Tokyo.[1] This article uses the term "triple disaster" for the 3 disasters combined. This triple disaster has highlighted the chronic shortage of mental health resources, which had existed in the region. This article outlines measures that have been implemented against the long-term impact of the triple disaster on scarce mental health resources, as well as mental health needs among the affected people and the state of mental health services both before and after the disaster.

BEFORE MARCH 11, 2011
Socioeconomic Status in Japan

The 2011 populations of Fukushima, Iwate, and Miyagi prefectures were 2,029,000, 1,331,000, and 2,348,000, respectively.[2] Younger generations have tended to move to cities where there are more job opportunities, and the Tohoku region is one of the least densely populated areas of Japan. As such, people in these 3 prefectures are older than in other parts of the country. In 2011, the percentages of people aged 65 years or older were 25.2%, 27.3%, and 22.4% in Fukushima, Iwate, and Miyagi, respectively, whereas the national average was 23.3%.[3] These 3 prefectures are more engaged in agriculture, forestry, and fishery than other parts of Japan. Among 2,605,736 Japanese people engaged in agriculture, Fukushima, Iwate, and Miyagi prefectures share 4.2% (109,048), 3.5% (89,993), and 2.7% (70,869), and these prefectures make up to 10.4% of the total share among all 47 prefectures in Japan. Fukushima, Iwate, and Miyagi prefectures are reported to contain 3.5% (11,322), 4.8% (15,685), and 2.0% (6397) of people engaged in forestry in Japan (325,589), totaling 10.3%. The numbers of people involved in fishery in Fukushima, Iwate, and Miyagi prefectures in 2011 were 1743 (0.8%), 9948 (4.5%), and 9753 (4.4%), constituting 9.7% of the total (221,908).[4]

The Tokyo Electric Power Company (TEPCO) owns Fukushima Daiichi (First) and Fukushima Daini (Second) nuclear power plants, which generate 4,700,000 and 4,400,000 kW, respectively. The total production of TEPCO's nuclear power plants constitutes 28% of the total power for 7 prefectures[5] including the Tokyo metropolitan area but, interestingly, excluding Fukushima prefecture. At the time of the disaster, the Fukushima Daiichi and Daini plants employed 1053 and 707 full-time workers, respectively.[6]

Pre-Event State of Mental Health

Needs

In 2009, Japan's suicide rate was 24.9 per 100,000, whereas the suicide rate of the United States was 11.3 per 100,000 in 2007 (age-adjusted).[7,8] However, higher suicide rates have been reported in Fukushima and Iwate, and seasonal increases in depression have been reported in the region.[9] The Tohoku region is a traditional rural area, and stigma attached to seeking mental health services is common, as in rural areas of other countries. In these areas it is difficult for local people, who have known each other since birth, to access mental health care and for mental health professionals to assess their needs, out of concern that their neighbors or coworkers might find out that they have mental problems.[10,11] It is relatively common for people to take a 2- to 3-hour bus or train ride to visit a university hospital for psychiatric treatment.

Services and system for mental health delivery

In the affected prefectures of the Tohoku region, there was already a severe lack of mental health resources before the disasters, such as lack of employment for mental health professionals and lack of accessibility to services, especially in the sparsely populated coastal areas.[10] It has been reported as of December 2008 that there are only 8.9 psychiatrists per 100,000 people in Iwate prefecture, with 9.9 in Miyagi prefecture and 10.5 in Fukushima prefecture, compared with 12.8 in Tokyo and 16.5 in the United States.[10,12] Although there is reluctance among older people to seek mental health services because of the stigma mentioned earlier, an increasing number of people who seek psychological counseling or psychotherapy has been reported across the country since the mid-1990s, owing to mounting socioeconomic disparities and interpersonal conflicts.[13] Despite such demand, lack of psychotherapy that is certified and insured by the government poses a further obstacle to care. No national licensing system has been established by a governmental organization to certify psychiatrists and/or clinical psychologists for psychotherapy or even psychological counseling.[13] At present, little or no coverage in the health care insurance system has been established for psychotherapy, although psychiatric medication is insured in Japan.[13]

THE TRIPLE DISASTER AND ITS IMPACT

The total amount of damage caused by the triple disaster is estimated at ¥16.9 trillion (approximately US$215 billion), including buildings (¥10.4 trillion), public utilities (¥1.3 trillion), infrastructure (¥2.2 trillion), and damage to agriculture, forestry, and fishery (¥1.9 trillion).[14] The tsunami destroyed coastal highways and railroads, which previously provided the main transportation system in the region, and prevented food and daily necessities, including drugs, from being delivered for the following weeks. In Fukushima people are still affected physically, mentally, and socially by the nuclear power plant accident. Rather than repeating detailed descriptions of the triple disaster's impact that have been already reported elsewhere,[9] the rest of this section differently describes the respective impacts of the Great East Japan Earthquake, the tsunami, and accident at the Fukushima Daiichi nuclear power plant.

The Great East Japan Earthquake actually comprised 4 magnitude (M-) 7 to 9 earthquakes occurring consecutively within a period of 40 minutes.[15] The first 3 epicenters, with M-9.0 at 2:46 PM, M-7.3 at 3:08 PM, and M-7.3 at 3:15 PM, were located within an area 200 km (125 miles) wide and 500 km (310 miles) long, close to the eastern coast of the Tohoku region.[15] The 4 earthquakes caused Japan's northeastern coastline to shift by as much as 4 m (157 inches) to the east[16] while the tsunami also transformed the landscape, washing away entire towns. Geophysicists estimate that the first M-9 earthquake accelerated the spin of the globe, causing the length of a day to become 1.8 microseconds (1.8 millionths of a second) shorter.[17]

Immediately after the earthquakes, a tsunami warning was reported by the Japanese media, estimating that the highest wave of tsunami would land within 30 to 70 minutes.[18] However, this was not enough time for many people to evacuate to higher ground, particularly those who were elderly, bedridden, or unable to take a quick action for other reasons. When the tsunami struck, some people were on their way to rescue other members of their family who did not have access to transportation, despite the ancient saying "*Tsunami, ten-den-ko* [Tsunami, self-evacuation]" being part of local wisdom. Some people managed to reach a local school (often one of the highest elevated buildings in town) in time, but were unable to enter because of the limited capacity of the shelter.[18] Others underestimated the seriousness of the warning and stayed in their homes. The tsunami was reported to be 17 m (669 inches) in height. The wave reached 10 km (6 miles) inland and 40 m above sea level (**Fig. 1**).[19] People lost family members, relatives, friends, classmates, coworkers, and neighbors. As

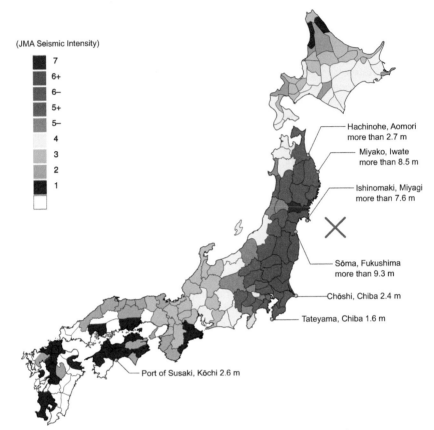

(JMA Seismic Intensity)

7
6+
6−
5+
5−
4
3
2
1

Hachinohe, Aomori
more than 2.7 m

Miyako, Iwate
more than 8.5 m

Ishinomaki, Miyagi
more than 7.6 m

Sōma, Fukushima
more than 9.3 m

Chōshi, Chiba 2.4 m

Tateyama, Chiba 1.6 m

Port of Susaki, Kōchi 2.6 m

Fig. 1. Map of Japan showing earthquake epicenter and seismic intensity.

seen in **Fig. 2**, the wave reached 2 m higher than the roof of the 3-story Disaster Prevention Center of Minamisanriku Town Hall, where the staff was working to warn residents to evacuate, sweeping away everything but its structure. Minamisanriku Town Hall has since posted a series of photographs on its Web site, depicting the impact of the tsunami on its Center building.[20] As **Figs. 3** and **4** show the devastating impact of the tsunami, many other photographs and video footage distributed on the Internet better depict the impact than verbal explanations.

As the major causes of death, 92.5% (12,143) of all fatalities (15,848) were caused by drowning, 4.4% (578) by compression under debris, and 1.1% (148) by fire, and 2.0% (266) were missing, presumed dead.[21] Before this earthquake, the Hanshin-Awaji Earthquake was considered one of the worst disasters when it struck Kobe and Awaji Island in 1995. In the Hanshin-Awaji Earthquake, 77.0% of a total of 6432 casualties were caused by being trapped or suffocated under debris, 9.2% were caused by fire, and 13.8% due to other causes, as of January 11, 2000.[22] There were 2.5 times more total casualties in the Great East Japan Earthquake than in the Hanshin-Awaji Earthquake.

The disaster had a particularly severe impact on older people in Japan. As of February 10, 2012, 19.1%, 24.0%, and 22.1% of casualties were reported to have occurred among people aged 60 to 69, 70 to 79, and 80 years or older, respectively,[11,21]

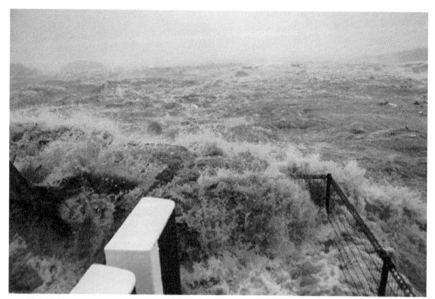

Fig. 2. The tsunami reaches the rooftop of the Disaster Prevention Center of Minamisanriku Town Hall, Miyagi Prefecture. Photo courtesy of Minamisanriku Town Hall.

indicating that approximately 2 out of 3 deaths were among people aged 60 or older (65.2%). In addition, the Ministry of Health, Labour, and Welfare (MHLW) in Japan reported that the Great East Japan Earthquake caused a drop in the country's worldwide ranking in average female life expectancy, falling behind Hong Kong after having been

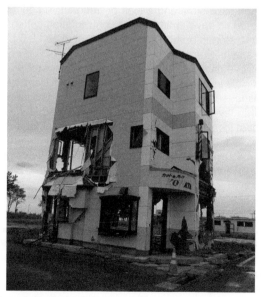

Fig. 3. A barber shop destroyed by the tsunami. Photo taken October 15, 2011 in Sōma, Fukushima by Jun Shigemura.

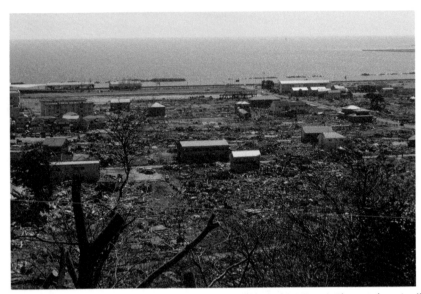

Fig. 4. A panoramic view of the coastal region in Ishinomaki, Miyagi. Photo taken April 1, 2011 by Jun Shigemura.

the highest in the world since 1985.[23] The tsunami may have had a particularly strong impact on this ranking.

Forty-six minutes after the first quake, a 14- to 15-m high tsunami reached the Fukushima Daiichi nuclear power plant, which was built on the coastline,[21] causing a third disaster for the people of Fukushima. This tsunami, rather than the first quake, caused a series of major incidents at the plant, including station blackouts, nuclear meltdown, a hydrogen explosion, and a leak of radioactive agent.[6] The radioactive-agent leak is estimated to have emitted as much radiation (when converted to uranium) as 20 Hiroshima atomic bombs and as much heat as 29.6 bombs.[21] The main leaked radioactive agents were iodine (^{131}I), strontium (^{90}Sr), and cesium (^{137}Cs), which have half-lives of 8 days, 29 years, and 30 years, respectively. Contrary to international opinion, officials in Japan had earlier reported the damage as level 4: "accident with local consequences," in accordance with the International Nuclear Event Scale, then raised it to level 5: "accident with wider consequences," and finally corrected it to the highest level, level 7: "major accident."[21] Serious contamination with radioactive agents was found in several cities and towns located within a radius of 20 km, and 70 km northwest inland of the plant. After the government reevaluated the evacuation zone, in light of the nuclear accident, on April 1, 2012, residents living in these areas were instructed to evacuate.[24]

The government implemented several safety measures for residents, such as monitoring the radiation dose within a radius of 20 to 30 km from the nuclear power plant, assisting inpatients to evacuate, and regulating food and drink contaminated by radioactive materials.[25] It is likely to take 30 years or more to reduce the radiation dose to a level that is safe for humans.[26] The plant shutdown caused TEPCO to concern about losing the ability to generate the power required by its service areas, which did not include Fukushima, leading them to implement rolling blackouts for the first few months after the disaster. It later became clear that the loss of the plant did not cause a serious lack of power supply.

MENTAL HEALTH IN THE ACUTE PHASE
Mental Health Needs

In the acute phase, inpatients needed to be evacuated from the mental health facilities that were isolated in the affected area. Continued care was urgently required, including the administration of regularly prescribed medication to people with preexisting psychiatric disorders. Cases of withdrawal symptoms due to drug interruptions were often observed.[11] In addition, many staff had to leave hospitals and clinics in the areas within a 20- to 30-km radius around the Fukushima Daiichi nuclear power plant, because of an inability partially to obtain correct information about the risk of exposure and partially to help reduce the extreme level of psychological stress.[18,27]

Thus, most people in the area experienced 3 traumatic events and were evacuated to shelters. Evacuees at shelters were typically cooperative and considerate to each other for the first few weeks, but later became exhausted as a result of not knowing when the situation would improve and feeling stressed about sharing limited space and resources with others.[1,9,11,21] The food supply was sometimes insufficient or inappropriate (eg, food that was close to expiration dates[18]), and stress caused by a change of environment may have triggered behavioral problems in the demented elderly.[11] As a result, evacuees were observed to become increasingly intolerant of the behavior of others at shelters. In the daytime people at shelters tended not to share their emotions, but at nighttime some privately wept.[10,21]

Across the 3 affected prefectures, at least 496 elderly patients and 82 nursing facility staff were killed.[18] Some caregivers were criticized by family members of elderly patients for not saving them from the mortal tsunami while other patients were rescued.[18] The psychological and physical burdens on caregivers supporting people with dementia increased as a result of decreased resources and deteriorated work environments, likely affecting the mental health of caregivers themselves.

Acute stress disorder, panic disorder, delirium, and psychotic excitement were observed among evacuees at shelters.[28] Others reported that evacuees experienced sleeping problems and anxiety.[9] Wandering and delirium were observed among elderly individuals with dementia because care services could not be provided after the disaster.[29] At this point, cases of serious acute stress reactions, major depressive disorder (MDD), or posttraumatic stress disorder (PTSD) were not reported at local hospitals and clinics.[9,29]

As in many places around the world, residents in the affected areas faced stigma of receiving traditional psychiatric treatment.[9] Many psychiatrists, working in a mental health team, were perplexed to observe little help-seeking behavior or verbalization from those who were affected, which differed from the everyday practice at their offices.[10] People at shelters were reported to exhibit "a restrained manner of behavior,"[28(p541)] avoiding the expression of negative feelings in the presence of others. After the Hanshin-Awaji Earthquake, mental health care professionals developed the euphemistic term *kokoro-no-care* (care of the mind) to avoid the negative associations with psychiatric treatment/intervention.[9] Some public health teams came to realize the usefulness of simple activities, such as measuring residents' blood pressures, holding festivals/tea socials, and providing classes for exercise, as nonverbal methods of identifying people in need of mental health treatment.[10]

Mental Health Response in the Aftermath

The MHLW established a central disaster response headquarters to better communicate with the local headquarters in Fukushima, Iwate, and Miyagi prefectures and thus take urgent measures for the disaster, including health and mental health issues.[25] In the early stages following the disaster, it was difficult to understand the details of events in the affected areas because of disruption to telecommunication and transportation systems.[28] Two days after the quake, the MHLW investigated the capacity of neighboring general hospitals, including psychiatric clinics, to admit new inpatients from existing facilities in the affected areas.[28] The MHLW dispatched approximately 380 Disaster Medical Assistance Teams (DMATs), which were locally trained to assist hospitals in case of emergency in Japan, to the coastal areas of the affected prefectures. DMATs conducted rescue work, and transported inpatients at hospitals isolated by the tsunami in collaboration with Japan Self-Defense Forces.[25,30] Transportation of inpatients was completed within the first week.[9] DMATs also attended daily conferences to share information and discuss what responsibilities to take at individual shelters.[11]

Because of the destruction of highways and railroads as the main transportation networks in the coastal area, a new way of distributing medication was required. The Japanese Society of Psychiatry and Neurology (JSPN) advised the MHLW about organizing drug distribution to the affected areas.[9,28]

The JSPN organized a disaster response committee 2 days after the earthquake, and several academic organizations established a mental health care disaster response operation center.[28] Approximately 30 medical care response teams across the country were voluntarily registered via the MHLW to local governments of the affected prefectures, and the MHLW promptly scheduled weekly dispatch of mental health care response teams for requests from the local governments in accord with the *Saigai Kyusai Ho* (Disaster Relief Act).[28] The Red Cross in Japan is required to serve as a public institution during emergency, which is designated in the Act and the *Saigai Taisaku Kihon Ho* (Disaster Measures Basic Act), and independently dispatch medical teams.[28] Other mental health care teams were not initially registered but became involved in the dispatching schedule at a later stage. These teams voluntarily collaborated with each other to mandate responsibility over certain districts.[28] For example, one distant prefecture sent out one medical team (eg, a psychiatrist, nurses, and a pharmacist) and one public health assistance team (eg, public health nurses and others) together. The public health assistance team visited shelters to conduct health monitoring and reported cases that required action by the medical team.[25,29] The main task of such a medical team was to provide on-site treatment and regular medication to people with preexisting psychiatric disorders, and to report cases of acute psychiatric symptoms.[28] Some of these public health teams also started temporary daytime care services at shelters, providing measures to detect behavioral and psychological symptoms of dementia among the elderly.[29] Because of the disruption of transportation and a lack of gasoline, medical team staff had no way of providing outreach services to certain shelters.[11]

MENTAL HEALTH IN THE POST-ACUTE PHASE
Socioeconomics

Although the rebuilding of highways and railroads has mostly finished, residents' lives, homes, work, and schools have not yet been restored. As of April/May 2012 in Fukushima, approximately 32,700 evacuees lived in temporary government housing, approximately 63,500 lived in private rental housing, and approximately 62,700 voluntarily evacuated outside of the prefecture. This evacuation situation has been unchanged since November 2011.[31,32] Many residents, particularly elderly individuals who were lone survivors, were left isolated after losing contact with their communities on account of relocation. In addition, a further lack of medical resources caused dysfunction among hospitals and nursing home facilities. Of the 139 hospitals in Fukushima, it is estimated that 110 were affected by the disaster.[31] Many people in the Tohoku region, who are self-employed or engaged in agriculture, forestry, and fishery, have been unable to resume working or to continue living normal lives. In particular, the consequences of the accident at the Fukushima Daiichi nuclear power plant do not seem likely to be resolved in the near future.[21] Distressing rumors about radioactive contamination by the nuclear power plant accident in Fukushima also keeps local agriculture and fishery from fully restoring their operations.

Affected individuals, particularly those forced to live away from their homes, are under stress because of an inability to see their lives recovering without financial support from the central government.[33] Following several evacuation policies after the disaster, residents have been either severely restricted from entering their households if located within a radius of 20 km from the Fukushima Daiichi plant, or recommended to leave or evacuate from their households if they are located in an area within which the cumulative radiation dose 1 year after the accident is expected to be 20 mSv or higher.[24] In the *Genshiryoku Songaibaisho Shienkiko Ho* (Nuclear Liability Services Organization Act),[34] the Japanese government admitted that it is socially responsible for nuclear damage because it promoted its nuclear energy policy, and allocated support mechanisms to TEPCO to provide compensation. It is reported, however, that TEPCO's dishonest response has tended to delay discussions on the compensation with numerous victims.[35]

Although some neighborhoods are excluded from areas designated by the government for emergency evacuation and have undergone decontamination, the current implementation of decontamination has been questioned. As of December 24, 2012, the local government of Iwaki city in Fukushima has started decontamination of residences, where the cumulative radiation dose 1 year is estimated to be more than 1 mSv, at the expense of the central government.[36] Nevertheless, affected residents are worried that decontamination of residential areas to the exclusion of nonresidential areas, such as nearby mountains, may only result in reescalation of radiation doses as observed in other areas already decontaminated, as well as in Chernobyl.[37] This means that returning home, as a symbolic act of recovery from the triple disaster, may not occur for the residents of Fukushima for some time.

NHK, the national television network, recently reported on the allocation of the ¥19 trillion reconstruction budget for the Great East Japan Earthquake, revealing that 26.6% of the budget has been spent on projects that appeared to be unrelated to the original intended purpose.[33] Lee Ielpi, the leader of the 9/11 Families' Association, argued on a recent trip to Japan that the bereaved in Japan should raise their voices regarding the unfair use of the budget and donations intended for reconstruction.[38]

Ongoing Mental Health Needs

No substantial increase in suicides has yet been reported following the disaster.[9] However, in July 2011 a 93-year-old woman who survived the earthquake and tsunami committed suicide in the backyard of her son's home in Minamisoma, Fukushima Prefecture, apparently because of stress related to the nuclear power plant accident.[39] In a note that she left behind, the woman wrote that she did not want to bother her son's family and had chosen to "take refuge in the grave." Her neighborhood had been required to evacuate immediately once it had been announced that the status of the nuclear power plant was likely to deteriorate.[39] Since a few months after the disaster, many people have perceived that they are going to lose their neighborhood support networks, and have diminished hope for the future without any concrete financial support provided by the government.[31] Given the long-lasting psychological effects of major disasters, it is important for suicides to be monitored closely from a long-term perspective.[9]

On October 3, 2012, the media reported that the local government of Fukushima had not made available an important piece of information regarding the health survey of cancer risk after exposure to the radiation, increasing suspicion of the government among the residents, including mothers with children or infants.[40] Exposure to radioactive agents is a serious threat to human life (both mind and body), even outside a 20-km radius around the plant, especially when the possibility of severe internal exposure to radiation through produce and seafood contaminated by radioactive material in the soil and ocean is still unclear.[21]

Nuclear power plant workers at Fukushima Daiichi and Daini reported perceived discrimination from their neighbors, who blamed them for the disaster, rather than treating them as postdisaster heroes.[6] Caregivers for the demented elderly have expressed mixed feelings regarding the staff members who stayed and those who returned after having evacuated.[18] Compassion fatigue and secondary trauma have been observed among Japanese mental health professionals and nongovernmental organization (NGO) workers.[11] It has been suggested that the mindset of many Japanese people in expressing *Gambatte* (which roughly translates to "hang in there" or "give it your all") to each other prevents them from taking steps toward appropriate self-care (Linda Semlitz, MD, Tokyo, Japan, personal communication, August 2012). Because psychological and physical fatigue among people in the affected areas have been observed from 1 to 6 months after the disaster, monitoring for the development of mental health disorders is considered important.[9,10]

As time passes, it became important to train local community workers in public health outreach and to screen affected people to identify those who are at an increased risk of developing enduring psychiatric disorders, such as PTSD, later in the recovery stage.[9] Mental health providers considered that teams using a public mental health approach (eg, community outreach) were required from the beginning of disaster relief response, whereas teams consisting of psychiatrists and other mental health professionals are important at a later stage for treating the long-term effects of disasters on mental health.[9,11,31,41]

Post-acute Mental Health Services

Approximately 6 months after the disaster mental health care teams started to pull out of the affected areas, and it became necessary to resourcefully use limited local resources for mental health care.[9] In this period, the MHLW developed a recovery plan for mental health services so that individual local governments would start discussions about providing more appropriate care as part of disaster measures.[9,42] Guidelines published by the Inter-Agency Standing Committee[9] advise local mental health professionals to:

1. Establish an organization that takes care of overall mental health, including the psychosocial aspects of people's lives
2. Show an understanding of how different the levels of exposure to an emergency can be among the people
3. Respect local culture and confirm confidentiality

Local universities took the initiative in resolving the lack of medical resources, and outreach activities were treated as new measures for those who were relocated away from preexisting medical care facilities without transportation. Fukushima Medical University established a clinic to monitor residents, particularly the elderly, in the grounds of several temporary housing developments.[31] Psychiatrists at Iwate Medical University planned the following 3 measures for postdisaster mental health care.[41]

First, counseling facilities should be set up at local public health centers while offering health care outreach programs at each shelter. To this end the local university, hospitals, and public health centers have collaborated on setting up counseling facilities at several local health centers in the devastated area, along with the eastern coastline of the prefecture, and universities and hospitals located 100 km inland have cooperated to support them.

Second, public mental health interventions should be focused on invigorating new communities from a long-term perspective. Activities at a common room in shelters, temporary housing developments, or community centers, for example, aim to rebuild new communities by reconnecting people who are relocated from their old communities and work environments (eg, primary industries).

Third, in accord with preexisting psychiatric problems and damage caused by the current disaster, the psychiatrists at Iwate Medical University have categorized affected areas as 3 risk levels: *Kenko* (Healthy), *Kyokai* (Borderline), and *Shikkan* (Distressed), enabling appropriate decision making about interventions for individual areas. This categorization not only helps those at high risk (ie, the distressed group) to access mental health professionals but also prevents the borderline group from developing mental disorders, possibly by referring them to professional care early on, and can help to educate individuals in the healthy group in maintaining and promoting their health.[41]

IMPLICATIONS

There are several important lessons learned from all 3 elements of this disaster affecting the local residents of the Tohoku region, particularly the people of Fukushima.

What Could have been Done Better for Mental Health?

The MHLW and several academic organizations, including the JSPN, responded to the triple disaster immediately and efficiently.[9] A disaster response committee was established 2 days after the earthquake and a mental health care disaster response operation center was organized. During the disaster response, the JSPN communicated efficiently and directly with the dispatched mental health teams via Skype at the beginning, and via televised communication later.[28] Japan Self-Defense Forces responded to the disaster quickly enough to transport isolated people, such as inpatients left in medical facilities and those who weathered the tsunami on the roofs of buildings, and to distribute medication legally obtained.[25]

It has been suggested that Japan's disaster response efforts be improved by including postdisaster mental health measures in the national disaster plan and by subsidizing or reimbursing professional psychotherapy provided for evacuees (Linda Semlitz, MD, Tokyo, Japan, personal communication, August 2012). Based on cooperation between central and local government, mental health measures should be built systematically through the country's disaster preparedness plan.[21] When medical teams from across the country pulled out and initiatives were shifted from central to local government, there were difficulties and confusion in decision-making processes.[21] Several decisions about where to dispatch mental health support teams were made by several employees of local government. Because different mental health care teams provided separate and sometimes conflicting services in the same city, it may have been better for the central government to extend the function of the disaster response headquarters, with local government staff working on-site as operating bases.[11,21] To this end, educating employees of central and/or local government to acquire expertise in developing logistics for emergency preparedness is required.[10,21] In addition, continued communication among various bodies (eg, mental health teams providing actual services on-site and academic associations/institutes monitoring them off-site as headquarters) will be essential for those professionals to build shared understanding about providing consistent and coherent mental health care and ensuring humane conditions for survivors.[28] The government should also play a centralized headquarter role during the postdisaster recovery stage,[1,21] financially supporting on-site disaster measures by external parties.

Another area of postdisaster mental health that could be improved in Japan would be subsidizing psychotherapy provided by mental health professionals for evacuees through the national insurance scheme. Unsubsidized psychotherapy can discourage the willingness of evacuees to access mental health resources. Although the MHLW waived copayments for disaster-affected people to receive medical care for 1 or 2 years,[25] extending this to the provision of professional psychotherapy should be considered for evacuees who are outside the clinic, so that psychiatrists and/or clinical psychologists in disaster health care teams can provide care to people who are affected by a future disaster but are unable to afford the full cost. To do so, the Japanese government would need to review and examine the coverage of professional psychotherapy within the current insurance system and the possibility of establishing a national licensing system for psychotherapy. The government, then, could decide where to provide psychotherapy under emergency situations other than at the doctor's office, and how to subsidize or reimburse clients other than inpatients or outpatients. The insurance system would also need to consider which categories of people to insure, such as those with preexisting psychiatric conditions or preexisting trauma history, the elderly who may suffer from dementia or other disabilities, and schoolchildren (Linda Semlitz, MD, Tokyo, Japan, personal communication, August 2012).

Which Mental Health Needs are Most Important?

To detect long-term postdisaster psychiatric disorders, such as PTSD and comorbid MDD, it is important to closely monitor people recovering from a multiple disasters over a long period.[43] Several studies have reported that disasters can result in an immediate increase in the symptoms of PTSD, MDD, and other anxiety disorders beyond what would be expected from the lifetime prevalence of the 3 disorders (ie, 6.8%, 16.6%, and 28.8%, respectively).[44] Suicide risk needs to be closely and continuously monitored in disaster-affected people. Because of the stigma associated with obtaining psychiatric treatment, providing treatment at the appropriate time can be difficult. Various public health approaches may increase understanding about mental health treatment, and reduce social and psychological barriers to obtaining such treatment.

Local people without experience in disaster response outreach who worked in the affected areas of Japan commonly experienced secondary trauma and compassion fatigue because of a lack of skilled leaders who understood the importance of self-care for volunteers. As a result, some people were engaged in their regular jobs at the same time as in outreach volunteer jobs, resulting in severe stress, and in some cases abusive behavior toward clients. These responders need special attention from a mental health perspective.

Moreover, the psychological effects of radioactive exposure on the health of residents, as well as first responders in a disaster, are often more severe than the physical effects of such exposure. After reviewing the consequences of the Chernobyl disaster 20 years later, the World Health Organization (WHO) concluded that the most serious public health problem was mental health.[9] In addition, for the nuclear power plant workers discrimination shown against them is another psychological problem.[6]

Which Mental Health Services are Most Important?

The triple disaster in Japan has highlighted the lack of convenient access to mental health resources, which are chronically scarce in the sparsely populated and aging rural regions of Japan. Three recommendations for addressing this problem are provided here. The evidence and/or reasoning behind each of these recommendations is also discussed. These recommendations could reduce the burden on local psychiatrists of monitoring evacuees for long-term mental problems.

1. Public health teams, instead of mental health teams, should start outreach as soon as possible after a disaster, providing support to people who are still affected by the consequences of the disaster. Comprehensive health promotion including nutrition, exercise, and life support is essential for such outreach programs.[41] Regarding mental health measures, dispatching teams of psychiatrists in the acute phase of the disaster should be held back until the post-acute phase. Whenever a public health team reports a possible case of severe postdisaster psychiatric disorder, psychiatrists should then implement outreach with mobile psychiatric services.[45] This approach would help to increase the efficiency later in the post-disaster recovery stage in accessing scarce medical resources, and to respond efficiently to the demand for psychiatrists.[41] Local health care support systems can play an important role against stigma in successfully providing preventive psychiatric interventions for the elderly and the bereaved.

   In fact, psychiatrists at local medical universities in the Tohoku region have recognized the necessity of outreach activities promoting comprehensive health programs, including mental health care. The mind, body, social relations, food, and lifestyle are closely interconnected, and it is important after a disaster to establish holistic measures with coordination of life support systems. For example, a town hall has provided free postdisaster medical examinations to residents aged 18 to 39, and to those aged 75 or older. This examination automatically included screening for depression (eg, the Quick Inventory of Depressive Symptomatology).[41] As mentioned earlier, setting up a common room for residents at the community center in a temporary housing development has been found to be another good example of providing such comprehensive health programs.[41]

   Psychological First Aid (PFA) is not a clinical treatment but a public health approach. PFA is a promising approach to changing the efficiency of public mental health outreach at an earlier stage of disaster response, and reducing the burden of psychiatrists. Unfortunately, the sole example of PFA's application in the emergency response to the triple disaster can be found in mental health services provided by the Tokyo English Life Line (TELL), a registered nonprofit organization, supporting the mental health needs of the international community throughout Japan. TELL was established in 1973 as an anonymous and confidential English-language telephone lifeline in the Tokyo metropolitan area. In addition to its Life Line, TELL has expanded to provide professional face-to-face and distance counseling and psychotherapy, psychiatric clinics, neuropsychological testing, and various multiple outreach programs.[46] Shortly after the disaster, in collaboration with International Medical Corps, TELL trained its staff in the WHO version of PFA, who subsequently trained at least 450 individuals working for nongovernment and welfare organizations in PFA.

According to Linda Semlitz, MD, Executive Officer, clinical director of TELL, and a psychiatrist trained in the United States, using PFA was found effective in strengthening confidence and efficacy of aid workers and health professionals who were interacting with subgroups of the affected population. PFA enabled those aid workers to improve their understanding of normal responses of the disaster-affected people, to assess each subgroup, to identify postdisaster needs among individuals for various levels of support including professional mental health treatment, to identify resources needed, and to learn about the importance of self-care. TELL recommend the public health approach, because resources quickly become scarce after a disaster, particularly in mental health.

PFA is also advocated in the guidelines for postdisaster mental health services, disseminated by the National Center of Neurology and Psychiatry (NCNP), with an emphasis on "resilience and watchful waiting in the acute phase."[9(p3)] The guidelines also advise against the postdisaster use of psychological debriefing. Psychological debriefing[47] was once considered to be a largely effective approach, and was introduced also to Japan soon after the Hanshin-Awaji Earthquake occurred in 1995. However, the technique has been discredited in the literature in the following decade, and is now cautioned against in the Japanese national guidelines for postdisaster local mental health.[9,48] In spite of this, some Japanese mental health providers continue to advocate for the effectiveness of psychological debriefing in preventing the development of PTSD among people affected by a disaster.[9]

For the first time in October, 2012, NCNP provided 1-day workshops to humanitarian aid workers as well as mental health professionals, based on the *Psychological First Aid Field Guide*, which was translated in Japanese from the guide written by the WHO.[49,50] NCNP adopted this from WHO's *Psychological First Aid: Guide for Field Workers*[51] because, compared with versions written by other organizations, its simplicity does not require psychological and/or psychiatric expertise (Yuriko Suzuki, MD, Tokyo, Japan, personal communication, December 2012), and enables people who came to volunteer and provide postdisaster psychosocial support to learn it in 1 day.[52] The guide helps people who want to serve survivors immediately after a disaster to learn what to listen for when talking with survivors, how to assess them, what resources are available, where to locate the resources, how to connect survivors to the resources, and how to avoid compassion fatigue.

2. Ideally, psychiatrists can serve first as advocates of humanitarian relief to provide food to survivors in the aftermath of a disaster, then as primary care providers to take care of comprehensive health, and finally as psychiatrists to treat psychological health from a holistic standpoint.[45] Connecting relocated residents with their new communities should come first before intervening in mental health problems, because rebuilding the foundation of lives is more fundamental than medical treatment.[45] As an example, providing safe playgrounds for children who live in disaster-affected areas may be more urgent and helpful than treating their immediate mental health.[45] Schools, churches, temples, and local Rotary Clubs in communities promote strong bonds between people. Collaborating with these institutions may provide an effective way to reach out to people requiring mental health interventions in the long term.[45] Psychiatrists should work hard to train themselves in primary care under disaster environments.[30] At the same time, physicians who work in disaster response should also have knowledge about the psychological effects of a disaster on public mental health over time.[21]

3. Another way of dealing with the lack of mental health resources is to maximize the use of local resources. Training health care professionals who specialize in disaster medicine and/or disaster psychiatry is necessary to prepare for various

types of disasters, such as earthquakes, tsunamis, nuclear power plant accidents, or terrorist attacks.[11] For example, a local network of mental health practitioners who were already working as a support network for suicide prevention agreed to also serve as a support network in the affected area for mental health following the triple disaster.[41] Gatekeeper training programs for suicide prevention[53] could be used to train staff in screening people affected by a disaster.[41] Educating local students about basic disaster psychiatry before they serve on-site as mental health professionals, in addition to improving education for mental health staff, is an important step.[11,21] It is proposed that these subjects should be taught to students who are in their last year of study at schools of medicine, nursing, and other health care professions.[11]

There is currently no agreement in Japan regarding the best way of training and supervising mental health professionals. Setting up an organization that supervises NGOs providing mental health services, and assesses whether they are doing an effective job and doing no harm to their clients and their staff workers, might help to address this problem. Past experience of the Hanshin-Awaji Earthquake revealed that Japan faced a scarcity of health care resources, and that the nature of training needs to be improved, possibly by developing an accreditation system (Linda Semlitz, MD, Tokyo, Japan, personal communication, August 2012).

Relevance for the International Community

The triple disaster that occurred in Japan in 2011, and the subsequent recovery process, can provide valuable lessons for the rest of the world, particularly in the successes and failures of mental health services. Future mental health professionals, who may have an opportunity of serving an international disaster response team, should be mindful of local national disaster plans, if any exist, and local health care practices and systems for evacuees. The international community of mental health professionals can also help a nation (eg, Japan) to develop high-quality guidelines for training and supervising mental health professionals.

Psychological distress among the people in the Tohoku region has been prolonged because of delayed postdisaster recovery, which is common in many disasters. Japan's experience with 3/11 suggests that the incidence of PTSD and comorbid MDD should be monitored closely over the long term, as should be suicide in areas with higher baseline rates, such as Tohoku. That compassion fatigue among caregivers for the demented elderly and perceived discrimination against nuclear power plant workers needed to be addressed in Japan highlights how different forms of psychological distress can be particular to subgroups within disaster-affected communities. As described earlier, public health outreach targeting different subgroups of the disaster-affected community is effective in dealing with scarce mental health resources and in reducing psychological and social barriers to receiving treatment. This approach should be applicable to other disasters and other countries.

The Fukushima Daiichi nuclear power plant accident is still an ongoing disaster. The media have conveyed the extent of the impact of radioactivity to the rest of the world, causing the German public to vote against the use of nuclear power plants in their country. Other countries, as well as Japan, are concerned with the consequences of this accident, because it can affect anyone who lives near a nuclear power plant or who comes to volunteer, as we learned through the Chernobyl nuclear power plant accident. For example, it is reported that even 18 years after the disaster, MDD and PTSD are still elevated among male workers who cleaned up the Chernobyl accident between 1986 and 1990.[54]

Despite recognition of the usefulness in PFA, the public mental health approach remains to be systematically proven to be more effective than psychological debriefing, with data collected across different cultural settings and disaster situations. As such, implementing the PFA approach in use in Japan, along with the guidelines written by the WHO and/or the Inter-Agency Standing Committee, as emphasized by the NCNP,[9] may be a sensible approach and may have implications for how other countries manage public mental health in the acute phase of a disaster. If clear evidence is collected about the usefulness of PFA, the public mental health approach may be recommended for inclusion in the national disaster plan of Japan and elsewhere. Japanese mental health professionals in the field should take responsibility for conducting this research with the financial support of the government, for the benefit of the country and, possibly, elsewhere.

REFERENCES

1. Yamazaki H. Miyagiken no hisai jokyo to sono taio—Sendaishi wo chushin ni. [Disaster situation and its response in Miyagi Prefecture—Sendai city]. Japanese Journal of Geriatric Psychiatry 2012;23:169–72.
2. Statistics Bureau, Ministry of Internal Affairs and Communications. Todofuken betsu jinko. [Population by prefecture] 2012. Available at: www.stat.go.jp/data/nenkan/zuhyou/y0203000.xls. Accessed October 8, 2012.
3. Cabinet Office, Government of Japan. Heisei 24 nenban koreishakai hakusho (Gaiyo ban). [White Paper on aging society, 2012edition (Summary version)] 2012. Available at: http://www8.cao.go.jp/kourei/whitepaper/w-2012/gaiyou/. Accessed November 9, 2012.
4. Ministry of Agriculture, Forestry and Fisheries. III Higashinihon daishinsai kankei todofuken tokei data. [III Statistical data on prefectures related to the Great East Japan Earthquake] 2012. Available at: http://www.maff.go.jp/j/tokei/joho/zusetu/pdf/08_2406_p69-93.pdf. Accessed October 8, 2012.
5. Honkawa Data Tribune. Denryoku gaisha no dengen kosei. [Power configuration of power company] 2012. Available at: http://www2.ttcn.ne.jp/honkawa/4111.html. Accessed October 7, 2012.
6. Shigemura J, Tanigawa T, Saito I, et al. Psychological distress in workers at the Fukushima nuclear power plants. JAMA 2012;308:667–9.
7. National Policy Agency. Heisei 22 nen chuniokeru jisatsu no gaiyoshiryo. [Summary report of suicide in 2010] 2011. Available at: http://www.npa.go.jp/safetylife/seianki/H22jisatsunogaiyou.pdf. Accessed October 13, 2012.
8. Centers for Disease Control and Prevention. Final review, Healthy people 2011: leading health indicators 2010. Available at: http://www.cdc.gov/nchs/data/hpdata2010/hp2010_final_review_leading_health_indicators.pdf. Accessed November 29, 2012.
9. Suzuki Y, Kim Y. The Great East Japan earthquake in 2011; toward sustainable mental health care system. Epidemiol Psychiatr Sci 2011;21:7–11.
10. Suzuki M. Higashi nihon daishinsai go no choukiteki mental health shien stage eno iko ni mukete. [For transition to the stage of long term mental health support after the Great East Japan Earthquake]. Occupational Mental Health 2012; 20(Special issue):48–52.
11. Uchida T, Fukatsu R. Saigai haken, iryo shien report—Miyagiken Kesen numa shi karano report. [Reports of disaster relief/medical aid—reports from Kesen numa city, Miyagi Prefecture]. Japanese Journal of Geriatric Psychiatry 2012; 23:185–90.

12. Scully JH, Wilk JE. Selected characteristics and data of psychiatrists in the United States, 2001-2002. Acad Psychiatry 2003;27:247–51.
13. Grabosky TK, Ishii H, Mase S. The development of the counseling profession in Japan: past, present, and future. J Couns Dev 2012;90:221–6.
14. Cabinet Office, Government of Japan. Bosai Joho no page. [Disaster information page] 2011. Available at: http://www.bousai.go.jp/oshirase/h23/110624-1kisya.pdf. Accessed November 9, 2012.
15. Jiji Press Ltd. Zukai, shakai—higashi nihon daishinsai, shingen iki to yosin bunpu. [Illustration, society - the Great East Japan Earthquake, epicenter zone and aftershock region] 2011. Available at: http://www.jiji.com/jc/v?p=ve_soc_jishinhigashinihon20110313j-06-w440. Accessed October 1, 2012.
16. European Space Research Institute. Mapping Japan's changed landscape from space 2011. Available at: http://www.esa.int/esaMI/ESRIN_SITE/SEMY4M0U5LG_0.html. Accessed October 1, 2012.
17. National Geographic. Daijishin de ichinichi ga tanshuku, jiku no shindo mo henka. [The earthquake shortened a day and changed the axis vibration]. In: National Geographic news; 2011. Available at: http://www.jiji.com/jc/v?p=ve_soc_jishinhigashinihon20110313j-06-w440. Accessed October 1, 2012.
18. Kato S, Abe T, Yabuki, et al. Hisai sha shien katsudo—Care staff no katsudo report. [Assistance activities for victims—reports from care staff activities]. Japanese Journal of Geriatric Psychiatry 2012;23:195–8.
19. Honkawa Data Tribune. Higashinihon daishinsai de kakunin sareta tsunami no takasa. [Heights of the tsunami identified in the Great East Japan Earthquake] 2012. Available at: http://www2.ttcn.ne.jp/honkawa/4363b.html. Accessed October 7, 2012.
20. Minamisanriku Town Hall. Minamisanriku machiyakuba bousai taisaku chosha okujo kara satsueishita tsunami no jokyo shashin. [Photographs of the tsunami taken from the roof of Disaster Prevention Measures Building of Minamisanriku Town Hall] 2011. Available at: http://www.town.minamisanriku.miyagi.jp/modules/gyousei/index.php?content_id=262 (for actual photographs: http://www.town.minamisanriku.miyagi.jp/uploads/photos1/2064.pdf). Accessed October 14, 2012.
21. Fukatsu R, Uchida T. Higashi nihon daisinnsai towa—Hakyoku no fuchi kara kibo he. [What is the Great East Japan Earthquake—From the depth of catastrophe to hope]. Japanese Journal of Geriatric Psychiatry 2012;23:143–9.
22. Hyogo Prefectural Government. Jinkodotaitokei kara mita Hanshin Awaji Daishinsai niyoru shibo no jokyo. [Demographic statistics of deaths after the Great Hanshin-Awaji Earthquake]. 2006. Available at: http://web.pref.hyogo.jp/wd33/documents/000036553.pdf. Accessed November 3, 2012.
23. Ministry of Health, Labour, and Welfare. Heikin jumyo no kokusai hikaku. [International comparison of life expectancy] 2012. Available at: http://www.mhlw.go.jp/toukei/saikin/hw/life/life11/dl/life11-04.pdf. Accessed October 1, 2012.
24. Japan Atomic Energy Relations Organization. Tokyo denryoku—Fukushima Daiichi genshiryoku hatsudensho jiko: Hinan ni tsuite. [Tokyo Electric Power Company—Accident at the Fukushima Daiichi Nuclear Power Plant: regarding evacuation] 2012. Available at: http://www.jaero.or.jp/data/02topic/fukushima/effect/evacuation.html. Accessed October 15, 2012.
25. Saito T, Kunimitsu A. Public health response to the combined Great East Japan Earthquake, tsunami and nuclear power plant accident: perspective from the Ministry of Health, Labour, and Welfare of Japan. Western Pac Surveill Response J 2011;2:1–3.

26. Japan Press Network. Jumin 15man nin wo 30 nen ijo kensa e genpatsu de ken-kyukikan. [Research institutes on the nuclear power plant accident to check 150,000 residents for over 30 years]. In: 47NEWS. Japan Press Network; 2011. Available at: http://www.47news.jp/CN/201105/CN2011051101001009.html. Accessed November 22, 2012.

27. Tago H, Kanno T, Amou M, et al. Fukushimaken no hisai jokyo to sono taio—hisai byoin no genba kara. [Disaster situation and its response in Fukushima Prefecture—from a hospital in the affected area]. Japanese Journal of Geriatric Psychiatry 2012;23:178–80.

28. Kim Y. Great East Japan Earthquake and early mental-health-care response. Psychiatry Clin Neurosci 2011;65:539–48.

29. Yatabe Y, Fujise N, Ikeda M. Saigai haken, iryo shien report—Miyagiken Minami-sanriku cho karano report. [Reports of disaster relief/medical aid—reports from Minamisanriku town, Miyagi Prefecture]. Japanese Journal of Geriatric Psychiatry 2012;23:181–4.

30. Sato S, Kodama M. Miyagiken no hisai jokyo to sono taio. [Disaster situation and its response in Miyagi Prefecture]. Japanese Journal of Geriatric Psychiatry 2012;23:165–8.

31. Kobayashi N, Niwa S. Fukushimaken no hisai jokyo to sono taio. [Disaster situation and its response in Fukushima Prefecture]. Japanese Journal of Geriatric Psychiatry 2012;23:173–7.

32. Kawahoku Shinposha. Fukushima hinanshasu, kasetsu ni 97,599 nin, yoka genzai. [Number of evacuees in Fukushima Prefecture, 97,599 people in temporary housing, as of 8th] 2012. Available at: http://www.kahoku.co.jp/spe/spe_sys1090/20120512_02.htm. Accessed December 1, 2012.

33. NHK Broadcasting. Higashinihon Daishinsai "Tsuiseki, Fukko yosan 19 cho en". [The Great East Japan Earthquake: "tracking the 19-trillion-yen reconstruction budget"]. In: NHK Special. Tokyo: NHK Broadcasting; 2012.

34. Ministry of Economy, Trade, and Industry. Genshiryoku hatsudensho jiko ni kansuru baisho nado ni tsuite. [Compensation and other concerns related to nuclear power plant accidents] 2011. Available at: http://www.meti.go.jp/earthquake/nuclear/taiou_honbu/index.html. Accessed November 12, 2012.

35. Yomiuri Shinbun. Genpatsu baisho, toden chien nara baishokin uwanose—shin-kijun. [New standard—additional charge into the damage compensation if TEPCO delays] 2012. Yomiuri online. Available at: http://www.yomiuri.co.jp/feature/20110316-866921/news/20120706-OYT1T01197.htm. Accessed December 25, 2012.

36. NHK Broadcasting. Jutaku josen Saidaikibo no chiiki de kaishi. [Decontamination of residences in the largest area started]. In: NHK News-Web; 2012. Available at: http://www3.nhk.or.jp/news/html/20121224/k10014394791000.html. Accessed December 24, 2012.

37. Tokyo Shinbun. Mienu josen, fushinkan, 3nenkan de 1cho en koka gimon. [Unclear decontamination implementation, distrust, trillion yen for three years, its effectiveness questioned] 2012. Tokyo Web. Available at: http://www.tokyo-np.co.jp/article/national/news/CK2012122302000095.html. Accessed December 24, 2012.

38. Ielpi L. The message from 9/11 disaster victims to a Great East Japan Earthquake victim. In: Suzuki M, editor. Symposium conducted at the meeting of Japanese Association for Emergency Psychiatry. Nara, Japan; 2012.

39. Yomiuri Shinbun. "Ohaka ni hinan shimasu."—Minamisoma no 93sai josei jisatsu. ["Now I take refuge in the grave."—Suicide of a 93-year-old woman in

Minamisoma] 2011. Yomiuri online. Available at: http://www.yomiuri.co.jp/national/news/20110709-OYT1T00649.htm. Accessed November 1, 2012.

40. Mainichi Shinbun. Higashinihon daishinsai: Fukushima daiichi genpatsu jiko. Fukushima kenko chosa de himitsukai. Ken, kenkai suriawase, Honkaigou scenario tsukuru. [Great East Japan Earthquake: Fukushima Daiichi nuclear power plant accident. A secret meeting on Fukushima health survey. Prefecture, modifying the view. The meeting made scenario]. In: Mainichi jp; 2012. Available at: http://mainichi.jp/feature/20110311/news/20121003ddm001040029000c.html. Accessed November 22, 2012.

41. Otsuka K, Sakai A. Iwateken no hisai jokyo to sono taio—Koreisha no kokoro no care wo chushin ni. [Disaster situation and its response in Iwate Prefecture—Care of the mind for the elderly]. Japanese Journal of Geriatric Psychiatry 2012;23:155–64.

42. Ministry of Health, Labour, and Welfare. The outline of the third supplementary budget of the Ministry of Health, Labour and Welfare (MHLW) of fiscal year 2011. n.d, Available at: http://www.mhlw.go.jp/english/policy/other/budget/dl/3rd-fy2011-e.pdf. Accessed November 22, 2012.

43. Breslau N, Chilcoat HD, Kessler RC, et al. Previous exposure to trauma and PTSD effects of subsequent trauma: results from the Detroit Area Survey of Trauma. Am J Psychiatry 1999;156:902–7.

44. Kessler RC, Berglund P, Demler O, et al. Lifetime prevalence and age-of-onset distributions of DSM-IV disorders in the national comorbidity survey replication. Arch Gen Psychiatry 2005;62:593–602.

45. Katz CL. A long term perspective on disaster mental health: from the 2001 El Salvador Earthquake to the 9/11 Terrorist Attacks. In: Suzuki M, editor. Symposium conducted at the meeting of Japanese Association for Emergency Psychiatry. Nara, Japan; 2012.

46. Tokyo English Life Line. History of TELL. In: TELL; 2012. Available at: http://www.telljp.com/index.php?/en/history/. Accessed October 13, 2012.

47. Everly GS, Boyle SH. Critical incident stress debriefing (CISD): a meta-analysis. Int J Emerg Ment Health 1999;1:165–8.

48. Bisson JI, McFarlane AC, Rose S. Psychological debriefing for Adults. In: Foa EB, Keane TM, Friedman MJ, et al, editors. Effective treatments for PTSD. Practice Guidelines from the International Society for Traumatic Stress Studies. 2nd edition. New York: Guilford; 2000. p. 39–59.

49. National Information Center of Disaster Mental Health. Konnendo no katsudo naiyo. [Activities of this year]. 2012. Available at: http://saigai-kokoro.ncnp.go.jp/activity/activity02.html. Accessed August 27, 2012.

50. National Information Center of Disaster Mental Health. Shinri teki okyu shochi (psychological first aid: PFA) field guide. [Psychological first aid (PFA) field guide] 2012. Available at: http://saigai-kokoro.ncnp.go.jp/pdf/who_pfa_guide.pdf. Accessed November 27, 2012.

51. World Health Organization, War Trauma Foundation and World Vision International. Psychological first aid: guide for field workers. Geneva (Switzerland): 2011. Available at: http://whqlibdoc.who.int/publications/2011/9789241548205_eng.pdf. Accessed December 2, 2012.

52. Japan Press Network. Kokoro nimo "oukyu teate" WHO tebiki de kenshu hirogaru keshosuruga oshitsuke nai. ["First aid" to the mind too. Training in WHO guidelines spread. Listen to their talks but do not impose]. In: 47NEWS. Japan Press Network; 2012. Available at: http://www.47news.jp/feature/medical/2012/11/post-779.html. Accessed December 16, 2012.

53. Cabinet Office, Government of Japan. Gatekeeper yosei kenshu text. [Text for gatekeeper training] 2011. Available at: http://www8.cao.go.jp/jisatsutaisaku/kyoukagekkan/gatekeeper_text.html. Accessed October 22, 2012.

54. Loganovsky K, Havenaar JM, Tintle NL, et al. The mental health of clean-up workers 18 years after the Chernobyl accident. Psychol Med 2008;38:481–8.

Hurricane Katrina and the Gulf Oil Spill: Lessons Learned

Howard J. Osofsky, MD, PhD[a],*, Joy D. Osofsky, PhD[b]

KEYWORDS

- Disaster respone • Childhood trauma • Posttraumatic stress • Hurricane relief

KEY POINTS

- Education and training about immediate responses, including the field operations guide for Psychological First Aid developed by National Child Traumatic Stress Network and the National Center for PTSD Psychological First Aid, are important for all mental health providers of immediate and continuing services to assist children, adolescents, adults, and families in the aftermath of disasters.
- To sensitively help with evacuations and return to normalcy, responders must be trained to understand the culture and traditions of affected communities.
- If family members are separated during a disaster, it is important to try to locate them, provide information about their well-being, and connect family members whenever possible.
- With disruptions and devastation, it is important to provide knowledge about available resources, including information about mental health, using central databases and technology to aid in gathering and communicating information.
- It is important to emphasize the need for routines and self-care for both victims and responders in an environment that, with recovery, will reflect a new normal.

BACKGROUND ON HURRICANE KATRINA

Hurricane Katrina, which made landfall on August 29, 2005, has been described as the worst natural disaster in United States history. Louisiana, Mississippi, and Alabama were all highly affected, with Louisiana suffering the most devastation and disruption to lives. Over 1,100,000 residents of Louisiana, ages 16 and over were forced to evacuate to other parts of the state and regions of the country. The Louisiana Department of Health and Hospitals confirmed more than 1800 deaths in Louisiana in April 2006; 750 people were still missing. In October 2006, only 62% of evacuees had returned to their homes.

[a] Department of Psychiatry, LSU Health Sciences Center, New Orleans, LA, USA; [b] Departments of Pediatrics and Psychiatry, LSU Health Sciences Center, New Orleans, LA, USA
* Corresponding author.
E-mail address: hosofs@lsuhsc.edu

Psychiatr Clin N Am 36 (2013) 371–383
http://dx.doi.org/10.1016/j.psc.2013.05.009
0193-953X/13/$ – see front matter Published by Elsevier Inc.

psych.theclinics.com

New Orleans Before the Disaster

Louisiana is a culturally diverse but poor state, ranking 49 out of the 50 states in terms of poverty, contributing to problems with the evacuation, family disruption, tensions between evacuees and receiving residents, and overall recovery.

The phrase often associated with New Orleans is "The City that Care Forgot" (Edward Larocque Tinker, *Creole City: Its Past and Its People*, 1953). This brings up a somewhat romantic notion associated with a sense of invulnerability and an acceptance of life, which may also include adversities with situations beyond one's control. Implicit in this fictional response strategy is the timing of response...slow and easy... things happen...all can be taken care of in its own good time. With Hurricane Katrina and, just a few years later, the Gulf oil spill, this existing attitude of many citizens changed because they experienced multiple adversities.

The reality of the situation in New Orleans and Louisiana preceding the devastation caused by these two catastrophic events is that many families were not faring well. Before Hurricane Katrina struck, New Orleans was a city that was both unique and typical. Its architecture showing a history of French, African, Spanish, and Caribbean cultures; its rich artistic history; and its location situated by lake, river, and delta were all one-of-a-kind. However, New Orleans also provided an example of patterns of segregation by race and by income that pervade many struggling American cities. Just before Hurricane Katrina, the US Census Bureau released a report on poverty in the nation that showed that Orleans Parish had a poverty rate of 23.2%, seventh highest among 290 large US counties. At that time, Louisiana ranked 49th of the 50 states on measures of child well-being (Annie E. Casey Foundation, 2005; Kids Count). Within the city of New Orleans, 30% of children were living in poverty (US Census Report, 2000) with two-thirds of families headed by a single mother.

The economic hardships in Metropolitan New Orleans were shared unequally. Although African-American residents made up 67% of the city's total population before Hurricane Katrina, they made up 84% of its population below the poverty line. In 2000, New Orleans ranked second among large American cities and far above the national average in its concentration of poverty. As poverty grew over the years in the city, middle-class families (including African-Americans) and jobs moved out, mostly to the surrounding parishes. Between 1970 and 2000, the city population decreased by 18% while neighboring St. Tammany Parish doubled in population. New Orleans was home to two-thirds of the region's jobs in 1970 but, by 2000, that proportion had dropped to 42%.

Hurricane Katrina revealed these disparities in stark terms. African-American and poor people suffered greatly from the devastation because, for the most part, they lived in the lower-lying, more flood-prone sections of the city, such as Mid-City or the Lower Ninth Ward. In fact, 38 of the city's 47 extreme-poverty census tracts were flooded. Unlike people living in areas of greater affluence that flooded, those in poorer areas had fewer resources, including access to a car. Racial inequalities and disparities were a fact that the nation and world observed during the evacuation period when so many individuals and families were trapped.

Children who live in poor families have frequently experienced more trauma than those in families who are more advantaged, placing them at risk for even more negative outcomes. The experience of the Louisiana State University Health Sciences Center (LSUHSC) Trauma Team and our experience with the Louisiana Spirit, the crisis counseling program, indicated that, in the immediate aftermath, in the many families who lost their homes and whose neighborhoods and were displaced, both parents and children appeared dazed or listless. Over time, families and children realized that the life they had come to expect with close-knit extended families and intergenerational commitment to occupations linked to the water such as fishing, was changing.

Impact of Storm on Infrastructure and Society

Hurricane Katrina's winds and heavy rains combined with the breaching of the levees resulted in 80% of New Orleans being underwater by as much as 15 feet, causing extensive damage to the city infrastructure. Individuals and families who were unable to evacuate—often because of poverty, lack of transportation, or places to stay—were sheltered and stranded in overcrowded hot shelters such as the Superdome and Convention Center. Supplies and information were limited with no cell phones or means of communication. Tensions, fears for security, and worries about evacuation and safety of families were heightened.

Hospitals, including mental health hospitals, were evacuated to the extent possible. Some, including Charity Hospital, the major public hospital, could never reopen. Damage to facilities, including those for medical student education and resident training, was extensive. Health and mental health education and services were severely disrupted. LSUHSC continued medical student education in borrowed, limited facilities at Louisiana State University while many faculty were forced to live on boats outside of Baton Rouge due to lack of available housing. Resident training in psychiatry and child psychiatry continued at scattered state mental health hospitals, Capital Area Human Services District, and via teleconferencing. When possible, because of the disruption caused by the extensive evacuation, outpatient services were offered in borrowed facilities. Tulane Medical Center students and residents, and many faculty, were temporarily relocated to Baylor Medical Center in Houston where education and training could be provided. Most New Orleans mental health professionals left the region and resettled in other parts of the country. Many did not return because of destruction to their homes, offices, and medical records, a reduced population, lingering deficiency in services, and the slow recovery of the community.

Several factors contributed to the many mental and behavioral health needs, including traumatic separation from family members and community, injury and death of family members and friends, loss of neighborhood stability and traditions, fewer religious facilities due to damage, and economic hardship with businesses unable to reopen. Often, one or more family members lost employment. People had to commute to devastated communities with few services for daily living. Further, there were increased workplace stressors and a disruption in education at all levels because most schools, colleges, and universities remained closed or needed major repairs. After disasters, schools often provide a secure base for families; however, the travel to schools and neighborhoods where they were operating often provided constant reminders due to the devastation. At the same time, many critical care and other clinical facilities remained closed or severely compromised. When care was available, it was provided in makeshift facilities that were just one more reminder of all that was lost. Fewer mental health professionals and public mental health services were available.

Soon after Katrina, the Louisiana Department of Public Health documented substantial psychopathology among 50,000 hurricane survivors in evacuation centers.[1] Household needs assessment surveys showed that half of adults still living in New Orleans after the hurricane demonstrated evidence of psychological distress. Across the state, in communities that were inundated with evacuees, tensions intensified because traffic and crowding become worse. The receiving communities became overpopulated, classroom size increased when schools assimilated the evacuees, and resources were often scarce. Increased stress and anxiety levels resulted from families and community agencies taking evacuees into their homes and facilities for protracted periods of time. The availability of Federal Emergency Management Agency (FEMA) trailers, although relieving the housing problem for many individuals and families, often created new stressors from living in cramped quarters with larger families and little privacy.

ACUTE MENTAL HEALTH IMPACT OF HURRICANE KATRINA AND THE DEEPWATER HORIZON EXPLOSION AND INCIDENT (GULF OIL SPILL)

To describe the acute and aftermath mental health issues, it is important to understand the backdrop for current problems. Louisiana is a poor state with limited resources, many heavily populated parts of which were devastated by Hurricane Katrina. Given its location bordering on the Gulf of Mexico, the state has been subjected to many disasters before and after Hurricane Katrina, including erosion of wetlands and other protective factors. The mental health concerns were then exacerbated by the Gulf oil spill. Recovery has been progressive, but incomplete, with mental health symptoms being persistent or easily reawakened.

In the week following Hurricane Katrina, the Department of Psychiatry at LSUHSC partnered with the Louisiana Health and Human Services Office of Mental Health Crisis Counseling Program and the Specialized Crisis Counseling Services (SCCS) Program, Louisiana Spirit. This partnership was designed to assist directly survivors with mental and behavioral health issues, specifically related to the stress and anxiety they experienced being displaced from or returning to devastated areas. Author Howard J. Osofsky (HJO) was appointed Clinical Director and author Joy D. Osofsky (JDO) was appointed Clinical Director for Child and Adolescent services for Louisiana Spirit. We, with other LSUHSC faculty well trained in trauma response, provided training and ongoing consultation for crisis counselors, specialized crisis counselors, peer counselors for first responders, schools and preschools, and traditional and nontraditional mental health providers. Working with FEMA, Substance Abuse and Mental Health Services Administration (SAMHSA), and the US Public Health Service, HJO and JDO and one other faculty member established and lived with a community on leased cruise ships to reunite first responders and city workers with displaced families and children. We also worked to integrate SAMHSA-recruited volunteers and Red Cross teams with communities in need of mental and behavioral health services. The Crisis Counseling Assistance and Training Program's Regular Services Program made 194,149 contacts with individuals. The greatest numbers of referrals were for disaster services, followed by other crisis counseling services, mental health services, and substance abuse treatment. Encounters included individual in-home contacts, brief educational contacts in home and group or public education settings. There were a high number of subsequent visits following the initial contact, reflecting the high degree of need expressed by the survivors and recognized by the outreach workers.

The SCCS Program conducted 4090 assessment interviews and follow-up assessments with adults significantly affected in Katrina-declared regions. The assessments showed that most adults receiving SCCS services reported experiencing three or more event reactions, including depression, sleep disturbance, difficulty concentrating, irritability, unwanted memories and nightmares, concerns about their ability to overcome problems, and reactions that interfered with relationships and physical health. Many survivors reported that the recovery was more stressful than the initial trauma, with ongoing challenges of housing, unemployment, and financial hardships.

Using a panel design with high retention rates, Kessler and colleagues[2] showed that frequency and severity of mental health symptoms increased, whereas use of services and prescribed medications deceased. Residents perceived mental health services and medications as less available and affordable.[3] In surveys of first responders from 2006 to 2007, including the Posttraumatic Stress Disorder Checklist (PCL-Civilian Version) and the Center for Epidemiology Depression Screen, over 40% of the first responders reported a desire for mental and behavioral health services for themselves and their families. The trauma team at LSUHSC Department of Psychiatry found persistently elevated symptoms of posttraumatic stress disorder and depression, as well as increased use of alcohol and partner conflict.[4]

In collaboration with LSUHSC Department of Psychiatry, schools in highly affected parishes administered over 25,000 assessments between 2005 and 2010 using the National Child Traumatic Stress Network (NCTSN) Hurricane Assessment and Referral Tool,[5] modified by school personnel, parents, and students for cultural sensitivity.[6,7] Forty-five percent of persons accessed reported posttraumatic stress symptoms and depression that met the cut-off for mental health services from 2005 to 2006 and 30% met the cut-off from 2006 to 2007. Although the percentage who met the cut-off gradually decreased during the first 2 years of recovery, it then plateaued somewhat in 2008 after Hurricane Gustav and the mandatory evacuation. In 2009, the percentage of students meeting the cut-off remained elevated compared with predicted after-disaster levels. This was attributed to the slow recovery, continued difficulties in reunion with families and friends, and persistent traumatic reminders from the extent of the devastation, as well as local and national economic concerns. To decrease the stigma of receiving mental health services and to increase accessibility, the LSUHSC trauma team provided training and consultation in providing therapeutic and supportive services to individuals and groups in schools. Students, their families, and the schools benefitted from these services. The authors' findings demonstrated that most students reported resilience even when they continued to have some symptoms.

THE LONGER-TERM MENTAL HEALTH IMPACT OF HURRICANE KATRINA AND GULF OIL SPILL

After Hurricane Katrina, in the authors' assessments, the risk factors contributing to mental health problems included damage to homes, belongings, and community; evacuation with little or no time to prepare; prolonged displacements from home; prolonged separations for families; unemployment and other financial losses; and additional traumas. The Deepwater Horizon oil spill, with its cumulative trauma and multiple risk factors, has played an important role because so many individuals, families, and communities affected were still recovering from Hurricane Katrina and other disasters. Although portions of parishes (counties) adjacent to the Gulf coast were more directly affected economically, the impact was widespread within families, friends, and communities. Families with intergenerational ties to the Gulf coast who depended on fishing wondered about the future for themselves and generations to come. Those employed by the oil industry, while anxious about drilling and safety, also needed to work to support their families in the only ways they knew how. They were concerned about how they would survive with the moratorium and decreases in drilling, and some of them worried about how to gain new skills and the necessity to move away to support their families.

Given this context, common adverse reactions included irritability and anger, distrust of authorities, uncertainty about the future, loss of enjoyment in life, all of which contributed to reactions that interfered with relationships and disrupted families. Many people found themselves having difficulty making decisions, sleep problems, fatigue, fearfulness, concerns about ability to overcome problems, and physical health issues. A common symptom was depression, including hopelessness, anxiety, intrusive memories and nightmares, and difficulty concentrating. They and their families reported increased use of alcohol and drugs including medications prescribed to themselves or others. A community leader expressed much concern that the initial symptoms represented the tip of the iceberg with greater symptoms yet to come.

It is important in understanding the longer-term mental health impact to recognize that mental health symptoms were still present when the Gulf oil spill occurred. Massive disasters, such as hurricanes, earthquakes, tsunamis, tornadoes, flooding, and fires, physically and psychologically affect adults, children, and families. Damage includes physical destruction, loss of homes, property, toys, pets, and, for many, separation from or loss of family members and community. Disasters with slow recovery and multiple complexities (a combination of natural and technological disasters) can be especially difficult for children and families, resulting in acute and chronic psychological effects[8,9] that negatively affect the child's normal developmental trajectory.[10] Families in the Gulf region have had to cope with multiple disasters—first Hurricane Katrina, then, approximately 4.5 years later, the devastation caused by the Gulf oil spill—resulting in cumulative traumatization and the possibility for development of community corrosion.[11–13] Another example of the interaction of complex natural and technological disasters is the 2011 earthquake, tsunami, and nuclear fall-out in Japan. The initial earthquake and tsunami resulted in a severe natural disaster that was compounded by the technological nuclear disaster, resulting in immediate and long-lasting individual, family, and community impacts, with continual concerns about keeping children and families safe from nuclear fall-out.[14] Large-scale disasters (eg, Hurricane Katrina combined with the Gulf oil spill, and the Japanese earthquake, tsunami, and nuclear disaster) are particularly important to children's development because they affect the individual as well as multiple systems, including microsystems and exosystems, in which children develop.[15–17] Exosystems include family, community, and society. Larger societal issues can indirectly affect children. For children experiencing such disasters, their once-thriving communities, including homes, neighborhoods, grocery stores, and playgrounds, are no longer functional. Many children and families experienced multiple moves and changes in schools, separation from friends and family members, and much parental stress resulting from family disruption and unemployment.[6,14,18] Families affected by such disasters are threatened with severe economic difficulties, loss of traditional supports, and even their identities because they must learn to live and thrive in other communities often with fewer economic resources. For those communities living by the water and depending on fishing for their economic survival as well as their identity, the tsunami and nuclear disaster in Japan, and the oil spill in Louisiana have threatened the tranquil fishing and wildlife areas on the coast. Disaster data following the Exxon Valdez oil spill[12,19,20] showed the significant vulnerability of children over time with much impact on individual, family, and community identity. Long-term outcomes for young children who are still developing are still in question, and such uncertainties are common for all children exposed to a disaster with slow recovery.

Mental and behavioral health symptoms following technological disasters are similar to those following natural disasters, but also differ in important ways. In 2011, HJO summarized the studies of mental and behavioral sequelae to oil spills.[17] Since then, the authors and others have provided theoretical perspectives and data applicable to the oil spill.[16,21–24] Of particular relevance are data from the Exxon Valdez oil spill in Alaska in 1989. In both circumstances, there were concerns about the ability to rebuild and continue multigenerational ways of life. The Deepwater Horizon Explosion and oil spill (Gulf oil spill) occurred on April 20, 2010. The flow of oil was not completely capped until September 2010. The quantity of oil spilled and the area of the Gulf of Mexico that was affected made it the largest oil spill disaster in history. Many ecological, health, mental health, and economic concerns arose related to both the oil in the Gulf of Mexico coming ashore and to the use of dispersants to control the impact of the oil. In the months following the oil spill, consistent with findings of Palinkas and colleagues[13] and Picou and Gill,[20] fishing families and those working in the petrochemical industry described mounting uncertainty about the future and distrust of authorities and information being provided (similar to the findings following the 2010 Japanese earthquake, tsunami, and nuclear disaster). Reported mental health problems from qualitative interviews immediately after the Gulf oil spill included anxiety, depression, increased use of alcohol and drugs, family difficulties, and indications of the beginning of a corrosive community.[21] Increased numbers of children in highly affected areas met the cut-off indicating need for mental health services based on the disaster screen modified by LSUHSC Department of Psychiatry from the NCTSN Hurricane Assessment screen. There was an increase in requested services (**Fig. 1**).

ADULT PSYCHOSOCIAL NEEDS ASSESSMENTS

To increase the State of Louisiana's capacity to address the needs of the population following the Gulf oil spill, the LSUHSC Department of Psychiatry with support from Louisiana Department of Social Services developed and conducted a mental and behavioral health surveillance in parishes heavily affected by the Gulf oil spill. Phase 1 of surveillance was conducted from August to December 2010. The assessment included 697 purposive telephone and in-person interviews with individuals in the portions of the parishes most highly affected. The following measures were included:

1. A Hurricane Katrina impact index
2. A modified version of the Sheehan Disability Scale to assess overall disruption of life from the oil spill, resilience, and life satisfaction

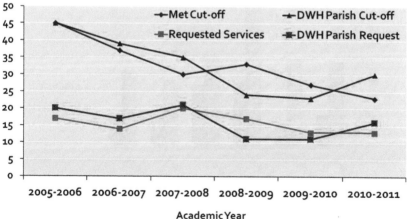

Fig. 1. Disaster screen modified by LSUHSC Department of Psychiatry from the NCTSN Hurricane Assessment screen showing increase in percent of requested services.

3. Mental health resilience (adapting two items from the Connor Davidson Resilience Scale), including the ability to adapt to change and to bounce back
4. Quality of life (from the World Health Organization Quality of Life Scale)
5. Mental health, using the K6 (General Mental Distress) to assess symptoms of serious mental illness, the Posttraumatic Symptom Checklist for Civilians, and Patient Health Questionnaire to assess somatic complaints.

Based on national standards, the results showed a high level of mental health symptoms. The greatest affect on mental health was related to the extent of disruption on participants' lives, work, family, and social engagement, with increased symptoms of anxiety, depression, and posttraumatic stress. Given that the location of the oil spill affected communities with previous devastation from Hurricane Katrina, results also revealed that losses from Hurricane Katrina were highly associated with negative mental health outcomes. Conversely, the ability to rebound after adversity and find satisfaction when reflecting on quality of life were highly associated with better mental health outcomes.[4]

Phase 2 of the adult surveillance received funding from SAMHSA Emergency Response Grant, Coastal Recovery Grant, and Louisiana Department of Health and Hospitals Office of Mental Health. Purposive in-person interviews with 1550 adults proportionally representing the parishes affected by the Gulf oil spill were carried out from June to December 2011. The Center for Epidemiologic Studies Depression Scale and Generalized Anxiety Scale were added in Phase 2. In addition to the symptoms already described in Phase 1, symptoms of depression and mild, moderate, and severe anxiety were elevated compared with national norms. The preliminary analysis of the effects of the oil spill on mental health symptoms comparing affected and unaffected portions of parishes is presented in **Fig. 2**. Reported quality of life was also directly related to the effects of the oil spill. A longitudinal follow-up with sampling of participants from Phase 1 and Phase 2 has been carried out. The results are not yet available.

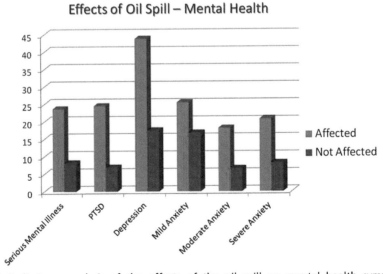

Fig. 2. Preliminary analysis of the effects of the oil spill on mental health symptoms comparing affected and unaffected portions of parishes.

RESILIENCE AND SELF-EFFICACY

Recent theoretical research has focused on examining patterns of resilience and recovery as it relates to developmental theories and trajectories for children. Important factors that support resilience in preparation for and following disasters include promotive and protective influences.[15,25,26] Masten and Osofsky[27] (2010) discussed promotive factors as those predicting better outcomes at all levels of risk or adversity and protective factors that are more important when risk or adversity is high. These two perspectives are extremely important in understanding the effect of disasters on children. The impact of disasters and developmental issues that follow are influenced by the nature and severity of the exposure; predisaster and postdisaster context for understanding disaster response and recovery; protective factors for positive recovery, such as strengths and individual characteristics; and, possibly, the child's age, and gender.[27,28] Pynoos[29] (1993) discussed factors that influence poor long-term outcomes following disasters, including extended periods of high cumulative adversity related to breakdown of infrastructure, ongoing economic consequences, family stress, loss of life and property, and other aspects of slow recovery.

Understanding how resilience and self-efficacy may operate in individuals, families, and groups following disasters can contribute a great deal to an understanding of responses and ways to support recovery. In the aftermath of disasters, it may be very difficult to maintain the crucial components of Masten and Obradovic's[15] short list that support resilience and contribute to individual self-efficacy. For example, with evacuations and displacements, families and friends may be separated owing to circumstances of the evacuation, including separations for reasons of safety, living in crowded shelters, and economic necessity. Further, parents are dealing with additional stresses, such as loss of homes, employment, and services, as well as uncertainties about the future. Other usual supports from community services are also frequently disrupted when caregivers, such as teachers, clergy, and clinicians, are also dealing with personal and community losses. These factors can interfere with effective caregiving and gaining support from family, friends, and community. Supportive schools and teachers are a protective factor; however, with displacement, children will often be in new schools with different teachers. For example, following Hurricane Katrina, children who evacuated from areas heavily affected by the storm attended an average of two schools with some children attending as many as nine schools in a year.[6,7] Faith and hope are important protective factors that can be significantly disrupted by disaster; however, with spirituality, this positive force for recovery is frequently present even in the midst of destruction following disasters. Self-regulation skills, another important protective factor for resilience and component of self-efficacy, are also frequently disrupted in the aftermath of disasters owing to the lack of routines, continual changes in living arrangements, school, and caregiving. However, for those children are able to adapt more easily, these skills are often present. For children and adolescents to show resilience and self-efficacy following disasters, there must be either some protective factors in place despite the disruption or confusion, or adults in the environment who, even with the uncertainty, can create a reasonable amount of stability and support.

To achieve positive outcomes, support from adults and an environment that creates a sense of normalcy despite the adverse circumstances are very important.[18] Although there is a great deal of literature on trauma experiences and negative mental and behavioral health symptoms, relatively little is known about how resilience following disasters or trauma contributes to a child's perceived ability to achieve future goals. The buildings of the St. Bernard Parish School System, about 10 miles from the city of New Orleans, were destroyed by Hurricane Katrina and the breaching of the levees. Personnel there intuitively knew that focus should be on disaster recovery as well as on the rebuilding of schools to help develop a sense of community and of future for affected children and their families. First, the authors approached the St. Bernard Parish Superintendent and Assistant Superintendent offices in Baton Rouge (where our team had evacuated and were working to find families as part of our disaster response). Later, in September 2005, we approached the second level of the St. Bernard School Administration Building (the first level was still covered with much and efforts were being made to start cleaning and rebuilding). At that time, most of the school administrators, principals, and teachers were living in FEMA trailers near the administration building and one remaining high school building where only the second level was usable. The St. Bernard Parish School Board opened the St. Bernard Unified School in temporary structures less than 3 months after Hurricane Katrina, becoming the first school to open in the flood zone in an effort to create a sense of normalcy for the children and families. The rapid planning and reopening of the school made it possible for many residents who worked at the school and in nearby factories to return and begin rebuilding their homes without having to send their children away to school. The LSUHSC mental health team worked hand-in-hand with the school when they reopened and continue to provide services for children and support to counselors, teachers, and parents in the now 11 rebuilt schools. The level of reported mental health symptoms, mainly posttraumatic stress and depression, were high in heavily affected areas and there was a need to develop creative ways to support resilience in children. To accomplish this objective, with funding from Baptist Community Ministries, the St. Bernard Unified School System collaborated with the LSUHSC Department of Psychiatry and developed the, St. Bernard Family Resiliency Project (SBFRP). This program was part of the school system's mission in promoting a positive and healthy recovery environment for their students. The Youth Leadership Program established as part of SBFRP has led to students developing helpful school, family, and community projects, as well as to demonstrating increased and lasting self-efficacy and leadership skills. Three years after Hurricane Katrina, in a longitudinal study of students in the St. Bernard school system, 72% of the students reported normal patterns of resilience; even those with mental health symptoms. Only 4% of the students reported patterns of breakdown without recovery.[7] The lesson learned from this remarkable public school system about the process of recovery following disasters is that rebuilding schools as soon as possible and school resilience programs are important parts of the solution.

MENTAL AND BEHAVIORAL HEALTH CAPACITY PROJECT OF LOUISIANA

The purpose of the Mental and Behavioral Health Capacity Project in Louisiana is to provide the urgently needed mental and behavioral health treatment and longer term supportive services to improve the overall well-being of individuals, families, and communities affected by the Gulf oil spill in Louisiana. There are similar and collaborative projects in Alabama, Florida, and Mississippi. The project is part of the Gulf Region Health Outreach Program under the preliminary agreement for the BP Deepwater Horizon Medical Settlement, with a grant to LSUHSC, with HJO and JDO as specified leaders. Target beneficiaries are residents in seven parishes highly affected by the Gulf oil spill with focus on the uninsured and medically underserved. In Louisiana, the project is focused in several areas:

1. Bringing integrated mental and behavioral health care to federally qualified clinics and other community clinics on site and via telepsychiatry, with the goal of increasing capacity and sustainability

2. Providing supportive and therapeutic services in collaboration with schools in these parishes
3. Training, consultation, and education for clinicians and community providers; to date, implementation has been successful.

Implications and Take-Home Messages

Preparation and training for disasters is essential but, by definition, it is not possible to be fully prepared for a major disaster. It is important to apply scientific knowledge to disaster recovery response so that environments can be created that provide the most sensitive support for individuals and families affected by disasters. It is also crucial that mental and behavioral health responses and support be fully integrated in overall disaster response to aid recovery and build resilience. Further, when supporting individuals after disasters, attention needs to be paid to past traumatic experiences so that increased vulnerability and risk are immediately recognized. Individuals and communities can and should plan and prepare in ways that will be supportive of children, families, and communities, and will promote resilience. Careful evacuation and relocation preparations need to be made that are mindful of special needs populations as well as keep families together.

All disaster responders, including traditional (police, firefighters, emergency personnel) and nontraditional (parents, community leaders, religious leaders, school administrators, teachers) first responders, need to be prepared to support individuals, including children and the elderly, two generally underserved populations, after losses and other unexpected traumas following disasters. In disaster response, mental health providers and others must collaborate with all of the institutions in the local community that will be in contact with affected individuals. To best support the recovery of individuals and the community, partners must include designated responders, volunteer agencies, hospitals and other clinically operational facilities, the faith-based community, police and sheriff's departments, school administrators, and teachers.

An important part of training and outreach is recognizing burnout or vicarious traumatization; that is, the process through which therapists' inner experiences are markedly influenced by empathic engagement with clients' trauma material.[30] This may have an impact on responders, even mental health providers, who work with and who are exposed to traumatized individuals. Individuals find their own ways to cope with these overwhelming feelings; regular support for individuals and by institutions is necessary, accompanied by self-care and reflective supervision if available. Mental health providers and other clinicians may have suffered from the disaster themselves and, therefore, may benefit from additional support.

The role of volunteers is important. However, their functions need to be thought through in advance so that they can be helpful and feel useful without creating additional burdens for local providers. With disasters, major disruptions occur in all areas and responders and helpers need to support establishing routines and, what the authors have called, the "new normal." This idea of a new normal has important cross-cultural implications based on our experience responding to disasters in other parts of the world. In disaster response and recovery, it is important to think out of the box and be open to providing mental health support in nontraditional ways while using learned skills to provide needed support. Being available and willing to listen is an extremely important mental health response. In the past 7 years, we have had the opportunity to learn so much about what can make a difference for those affected by multiple disasters.

Education and training about immediate responses, including the field operations guide for Psychological First Aid developed by NCTSN and the National Center for

PTSD Psychological First Aid, are important for all mental health providers of immediate and continuing services to assist children, adolescents, adults, and families in the aftermath of disasters. Responders need to be trained to understand the culture and traditions of affected communities to help sensitively with evacuations and the return to normalcy. If family members are separated during a disaster, it is important to try to locate them, provide information about their well-being, and connect family members whenever possible. When responding to disruptions and devastation, it is important to gather and communicate knowledge about available resources, including information about mental health using central databases and technology. Finally, it is important to emphasize the need for routines and self-care for both victims and responders in an environment that, with recovery, will reflect a new normal.

REFERENCES

1. Centers for Disease Control and Prevention. Public health response to Hurricanes Katrina and Rita—Louisiana, 2005. MMWR Morb Mortal Wkly Rep 2006; 55:29–30.
2. Kessler RC, Galea S, Gruber MJ, et al. Trends in mental illness and suicidality after Hurricane Katrina. Mol Psychiatry 2008;13:374–84.
3. Kaiser Permanente. Available at: http://www.kff.org/katrina. Accessed September 4, 2012.
4. Osofsky HJ, Osofsky JD, Hansel TC. Deepwater horizon oil spill: mental health effects on residents in heavily affected areas [abstract]. Disaster Med Public Health Prep 2011;5(4):280–6.
5. Hurricane Assessment and Referral Tool. Available at: http://www.nctsnet.org/nctsn_assets/pdfs/intervention_manuals/referraltool.pdf. Accessed November 5, 2012.
6. Osofsky H, Osofsky J, Kronenberg M, et al. Posttraumatic stress symptoms in children after Hurricane Katrina: predicting the need for mental health services. Am J Orthop 2009;79:212–20.
7. Kronenberg ME, Hansel TC, Brennan AM, et al. Children of Katrina: lessons learned about post-disaster symptoms and recovery patterns. Child Development 2010;81:1241–59.
8. Kessler RC, Galea S, Jones RT, et al. Mental illness and suicidality after Hurricane Katrina. Bull World Health Organ 2006;84:930–9.
9. Osofsky JD, Osofsky HJ, Kronenberg M, et al. The aftermath of Hurricane Katrina: mental health considerations and lessons learned. In: Kilmer R, Gil-Rivas V, Tedeschi R, et al, editors. Meeting the needs of children, families, and communities post-disaster: lessons learned from Hurricane Katrina and its aftermath. Washington, DC: American Psychological Association Press; 2009. p. 241–63.
10. Pynoos R, Steinberg A, Piacentini J. A developmental psychopathology model of childhood traumatic stress and intersection with anxiety disorders. Biol Psychiatry 1999;46:1542–54.
11. Picou JS, Marshall BK, Gill DA. Disaster, litigation, and the corrosive community. Social Forces 2004;82:1493–522.
12. Palinkas LA. The Exxon Valdez oil spill. In: Neria Y, Galea S, Norris F, editors. Mental health consequences of disasters. New York: Cambridge University Press; 2009. p. 454–72.
13. Palinkas LA, Petterson JS, Russell J, et al. Community patterns of psychiatric disorder after the Exxon Valdez oil spill. Am J Psychiatry 1993;150: 1517–23.

14. Watanabe H. The Manifold Impact of Radiation on Children and Families in Fukushima. Paper presented at The Great East Japan Earthquake and Disasters: One Year Later, Sponsored by the UCSF Departments of Psychiatry and Pediatrics and Global Health Sciences, San Francisco, March 12, 2012.

15. Masten AS, Obradović J. Disaster preparation and recovery: lessons from research on resilience in human development. Ecology Society 2008;13(1):9.

16. Osofsky HJ, Palinkas LA, Galloway JA. Mental health effects of the gulf oil spill. Disaster Med Public Health Prep 2010;4:273–6.

17. Goldstein BD, Osofsky HJ, Lichtveld MY. The Gulf oil spill. N Engl J Med 2011; 364:1334–45.

18. Osofsky JD, Osofsky HJ, Harris WW. Katrina's children: social policy for children in disasters. Soc Policy Rep 2007;21(1):1–20.

19. Lessons from the Exxon Valdez: Oil spills shatter relationships and communities. Available at: http://www.onearth.org/article/lessons-from-the-exxon-valdez. Accessed May 14, 2010.

20. Picou JS, Gill DA. The Exxon Valdez oil spill and chronic psychological stress. American Fisheries Society Symposium 1996;18:879–93.

21. Palinkas LA. A conceptual framework for understanding the mental health impacts of oil spills: lessons from the Exxon Valdez oil spill. Psychiatry 2012; 75:203–22.

22. Osofsky HJ, Osofsky JD, Hansel TC. Commentary: mental health perspectives following the Gulf oil spill. Psychiatry 2012;75:232–4.

23. Redlener I. 2010. Available at: http://www.mailman.columbia.edu/news/oil-spill-has-far-reaching-effects-children-and-families. Accessed November 5, 2012.

24. Yun K, Lurie N, Hyde PS. Perspective: moving mental health into the disaster-preparedness spotlight. N Engl J Med 2010;363(13):1–3.

25. Bonanno GA, Mancini AD. The human capacity to thrive in the face of potential trauma. Pediatrics 2008;121:369–75.

26. Layne CM, Beck CJ, Rimmasch H, et al. Promoting "resilient" posttraumatic adjustment in childhood and beyond: "Unpacking" life events, adjustment trajectories, resources, and interventions. In: Brom D, Pat-Horenczyk R, Ford J, editors. Treating traumatized children: risk, resilience, and recovery. New York: Routledge; 2009. p. 13–47.

27. Masten AS, Osofsky JD. Disasters and their impact on child development: introduction to the special section. Child Dev 2010;81:1029–39.

28. Masten AS, Narayan AJ. Child development in the context of disaster, war, and terrorism: pathways of risk and resilience. Annu Rev Psychol 2012;63:227–57.

29. Pynoos R. Traumatic stress and developmental psychopathology in children and adolescents. In: Oldham J, Riba M, Tasman A, editors. American Psychiatric Press Review of psychiatry, vol. 12. Washington, DC: American Psychiatric Press; 1993. p. 205–38.

30. McCann IL, Pearlman LA. Vicarious traumatization: a framework for the psychological effects of working with victims. J Trauma Stress 1990;3:131–49.

The Perspective of Psychosocial Support a Decade after Bam Earthquake: Achievements and Challenges

Ali Farhoudian, MD[a], Ahmad Hajebi, MD[b,*],
Ali Bahramnejad, MS, MPH[c], Craig L. Katz, MD[d]

KEYWORDS

- Disasters • Earthquakes • Bam • Psychosocial support • Grief
- Posttraumatic stress disorder

KEY POINTS

- In today's changing world, disasters like floods and earthquakes can have very different consequences in terms of depth and breadth, magnitude, and preparedness of society.
- Disaster can be seen as a consequence or manifestation of the lack of progress and development. A disaster is often a consequence of weakness and vulnerability of systems, not just the magnitude of the event.
- A crisis turns into a disaster when the society is not capable of properly confronting and managing a situation.
- Identification and definition of capability as well as recognizing the nature and extent of personal and social capabilities in a community are priceless in preventing disasters and reducing their consequent destruction.
- This article reviews the Bam earthquake, one of the greatest disasters of the last decade in Iran, and discusses its economic, social, and mental health impacts on survivors from the first days after the event and particularly its effects in the following weeks, months, and years.

BAM BEFORE THE EARTHQUAKE

Kerman Province is located in the southeast of Iran, with its capital the city of Kerman.[1–3] Covering approximately 11% of Iran's total area, Kerman is among the important and historical provinces of the country and is the industrial, cultural, political, agricultural, academic, and religious pole of the southeastern provinces.[4]

[a] Substance Abuse and Dependence Research Center, University of Social Welfare and Rehabilitation Sciences, Tehran 1985713834, Iran; [b] Department of Psychiatry, Mental Health Research Center, Tehran Psychiatry Institute, Iran University of Medical Sciences, Tehran 1445613111, Iran; [c] Kerman University of Medical Sciences, Kerman 7618747653, Iran; [d] Mount Sinai School of Medicine, New York, NY 10029, USA
* Corresponding author.
E-mail address: A-hajebi@tums.ac.ir

Psychiatr Clin N Am 36 (2013) 385–402
http://dx.doi.org/10.1016/j.psc.2013.05.003
0193-953X/13/$ – see front matter © 2013 Elsevier Inc. All rights reserved.

psych.theclinics.com

Before the earthquake, the Bam district (**Fig. 1**) had a population of approximately 240,000, among which approximately 97,000 were living in urban and 143,000 in rural areas. The average number of people per household was estimated as 5.85 and approximately 48% of the Bam population was below 20 years of age.[5,6]

Bam enjoyed a desirable economic and social status compared with its neighboring cities because of the presence of date palm gardens, a special economic zone, and the greatest ancient mud-brick citadel in the world, Arg-é Bam. It has a history dating back 2000 years and symbolizes of the cultural and historical antiquity of the region. The Arg-é Bam citadel was a major tourism attraction and many tourists from different parts of the world traveled to Bam to visit. The average income of Bam residents used to be 1,474,200 rials (1 US dollar was equal to 8800 rials at the time).[7] Precise statistics of the income and financial turnover of the area are not available; however, the economic significance of Bam are described.

Agriculture and animal husbandry played a major role in the economy of Bam. Orange orchards, palm groves, and farms covered most of the city. Other services included commercial, transportation, communication, and financial services (like insurance companies) and public and private services.[5] Due to the presence of the Arg-e Jadid special economic zone and the neighboring industrial city (**Fig. 2**), Bam used to be an economic anchor for Kerman Province and the country. Various industries, such as the automotive industry, oil refineries, and storage of agricultural products, were located in Bam.[5] Kerman Province and Bam were once among the most important illicit drug trafficking intersections from Afghanistan to other parts of the country and abroad, and it seems that drug trafficking plays a role in the informal economy of the area while posing an unhealthy criminal presence.

Primary health care had approximately 100% coverage of population in the city of Bam and its neighboring villages. Public health care and therapeutic services were provided via 13 rural and 15 urban health centers, 112 health houses, 1 health post, and 2 general hospitals. Psychiatric services were provided by a psychiatrist in the city, and a plan for the integration of mental health services in primary health care had been implemented in 80% of rural areas. Although rates of utilization are unclear, general mental health services, including patient screening, referrals, education, and follow-ups, were mostly done by trained individuals in the primary health care system

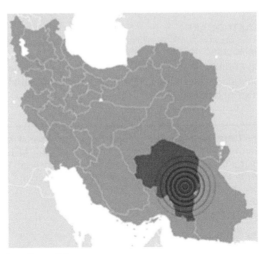

Fig. 1. Geographic location of Bam.

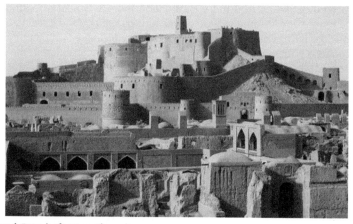

Fig. 2. Arg-é Bam before earthquake.

whereas other mental health care services were not provided systematically. Two important mental health indicators in the region were 22.8% prevalence of psychiatric disorders[8] and a suicide rate of 9 per 100,000 (Kerman University of Medical Sciences, unpublished data, 2003). In Iran, these indicators were 21% prevalence[8] and 6 per 100,000, respectively, at the time. Opiate consumption and addiction (mainly opium), a tradition for centuries, was common in Bam society at the time of the disaster.

THE EARTHQUAKE AND ITS IMPACT

The Bam earthquake was a psychological, social, and humanitarian catastrophe associated with serious economic side effects. The earthquake struck the historical city, Bam, and surrounding villages on December 26, 2003, at 5:26 AM. Its magnitude was estimated at 6.6 on the Richter scale (**Fig. 3**).

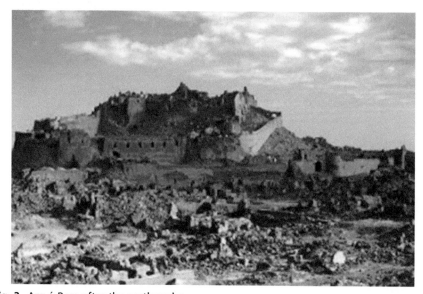

Fig. 3. Arg-é Bam after the earthquake.

The Bam earthquake caused more destruction than is typical of earthquakes of comparable magnitude.[9] Both the type of the earthquake and the building structures were responsible for the mass destruction of Bam earthquake. This earthquake was rare in because it affected horizontal, vertical, and inclined structures; the buildings in the region were often built in the traditional mud-brick style and could not survive such an earthquake. Approximately 20,000 houses, 100% of health centers, and 80% of hospitals were completely destroyed, and electricity, water supplies, and telecommunication were cut by the earthquake.

Widespread destruction of houses; the early morning timing of the earthquake, when most people were asleep; destruction of health centers all over the city that made helping the injured impossible; and a severe drop in temperature on the first nights after the earthquake all made the situation intolerable for the survivors[10] and raised the death toll.

The earthquake left approximately 28,000 dead and 30,000 injured.[11] Many writers, scientists, farmers, and businessmen; approximately 8000 to 10,000 students; 560 teachers; and 200 health care workers lost their lives.[12] In total, 37.5% of the populace reported having been trapped under the rubble after the earthquake, of which 81% escaped themselves whereas 29.4% were pulled out with the help of others; 17.4% had minor injuries and needed outpatient medical treatment, 14.7% were severely injured and needed hospitalization, and 3.1% were severely and permanently injured, needed amputation, or were paralyzed.[7] The earthquake left approximately 2000 widowed women, 1600 widowed men, 1200 children with no parents, and 3000 children with a single parent. Approximately 400 survivors suffered permanent physical disability. According to a study, 89.3% of survivors lost at least 1 first-degree or second-degree relative[13]; 89% of youngsters lost at least 1 of their parents.[14] Each survivor lost 1 to 40 relatives.[7] Bam citizens experienced the most severe stress of their life (**Fig. 4**).

Another consequence of the high-magnitude earthquake that compounded its impact was the rapid increase of urban population. Despite the high death toll and survivors moving out of the city, the population in the destructed area (city and village) reached 102,000 due to the need for workers to assist in the reconstruction phase.[11] High wages and the benefits of temporary shelters and other earthquake relief

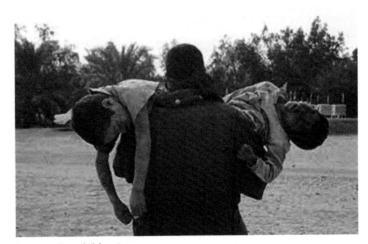

Fig. 4. Father carrying children's corpses.

services attracted people from the surrounding villages.[15] Most villagers had lived in surrounding villages that were untouched by the earthquake but were economically dependent on Bam. The death of a large number of Bam citizens along with the arrival of immigrants resulted in disintegration of previous social networks and formation of a new social network of immigrants.[2] Social relations, civic order, and communication networks were severely affected after the earthquake; 40% of people admitted that the earthquake had many negative impacts on their social relations whereas 24.6% believed that the earthquake increased the spirit of cooperation and unanimity and decreased animosity between local tribes.[2] An increased sense of possessiveness among the pre-earthquake citizens toward their city, job loss, and severe damage to social networks together with the loss of loved ones and personal assets, as in any severe earthquake, turned the Bam earthquake into a psychological disaster. In the first few days after the earthquake, widespread theft of personal property added to the sense of insecurity as outsiders streamed into Bam.

ACUTE IMPACT AND INTERVENTIONS

The National Commission for Human Development was established within hours of the earthquake by the Ministry of Health and Medical Education. This commission was responsible for health preservation in the affected area and assistance in coordination of services provided for district managers. After a rapid needs assessment, the commission defined its tasks as offering primary care services to the survivors in the form of public health training, environmental health, mental health services, counseling services, and providing for primary human needs, such as healthy drinking water, food, and portable restrooms.[16]

Vast activity in the field of psychosocial support in Bam began by the Ministry of Health on the second day after the earthquake. These activities included the following[16]: establishing a psychosocial support headquarters in Bam by a mental health office director; rapid assessment of the psychological status of survivors through quantitative methods; immediate reporting of missing relatives and coordination of reunions (from the first, Internet connection was established and made it possible for survivors to contact their relatives in other parts of the world); participating in the funeral and mourning ceremonies and rituals alongside the survivors; holding regular meetings for mental health care providers under the supervision of the Ministry of Health and with the cooperation of Red Crescent Society and the Welfare Organization; trying to attract human resources from different parts of the country; and, last but not least, supporting orphans and organizing them through the Welfare organization of the province.

The immediate needs of survivors included food, water, shelter, bathroom, restroom, heating and cooking appliances, and general safety and security.[10,17] By the second day, due to the high prevalence of opium addiction in Bam, opiate withdrawal syndrome gradually developed and assumed a place as a basic need.[18] Considering the dominant culture and family-oriented lifestyle of Bam citizens, knowing about the health and safety of relatives, reuniting with their family members, and recovering the corpses of loved ones and tending to their funerals were especially important. It seemed that in some cases, survivors assigned a higher priority to these issues than their needs for food, clothing, and warm shelter. Other needs during the first days included the desire to help with rescue and recovery services; concerns about the equal distribution of services; medical teams having appropriate understanding of what the survivors were going through; and the physical and mental needs of the aid workers.[17]

Unfortunately, efforts by the Ministry of Health to meet these needs in the first few days were insufficient and delayed. In the first 10 days, canned food and bread were the most widely distributed foods,[19] but 98.9% of the injured survivors were dissatisfied with the supply and distribution of food after the earthquake. Approximately 77.8% believed the quality of the distributed food was low, and 80.3% were complaining about lack of food variety.[19] One study revealed that 72.2% of the survivors assessed the aid in the first days after the earthquake as weak.[20]

The sudden influx of people who had migrated into Bam in the first days after the earthquake posed a problem for aid workers. Because these people were less injured, had not experienced losses, and did not suffer the shock of trauma, they were the first to receive aid and services. As a result, there was a shortage of resources when it came to afflicted people of Bam. The aid workers were incapable of differentiating between these people and survivors and gradually developed distrust of all those in need of help. A majority of survivors were satisfied with the system informing them about the status of their afflicted relatives in the acute phase of disaster but evaluated the role of media in organizing people and their appropriate reaction as moderate.[21]

Severe grief, anger, depression, restlessness, and hopelessness were among the most important psychological problems of the survivors in the first days after the earthquake. Most of Bam citizens were experiencing a deep grief due to loss of their loved ones and 75% of adults were diagnosed with acute stress disorder.[14] Acute stress symptoms were severe in 12%, moderate in 35%, and mild in 44% of children.[14] Symptoms of anxiety, depression, anger, posttraumatic stress, and dissociation were significant among teenagers.[14] Hopelessness about the future and anger was so severe that most adults did not welcome visits from authorities.[21] Some survivors even became suspicious of them. For example, many believed that no earthquake had occurred and that the tremors and destruction were due to underground military experiments. Meanwhile, others thought the earthquake was God's revenge because of their sins (especially substance abuse) and felt guilt and anger toward themselves or their relatives.

Because most physicians and nurses had not received adequate training for management of patients with drug dependence,[18] they were not successful in adequately controlling the withdrawal symptoms in opioid-dependent patients. Although approximately half of the opioid-dependent people talked to the health care workers about their problem and asked for sedatives and narcotics, withdrawal symptoms were controlled by administration of narcotics in only one-fourth and more than two-thirds had to use opium.[22] Thus, from the beginning, use of narcotics was expected to increase among the survivors.[23] Homelessness, unemployment, and probably greater demand for illicit drugs led to a surge in the drug market as the price of illegal substances went up.[24]

Considering all these factors, the authors realized that survivors' mental health was among the most important concerns of the psychosocial support headquarters. Extensive outreach and tent visits by trained psychologists and psychiatrists constituted the main activities in the acute phase after the disaster. First, they initiated psychosocial support, psychological debriefing (an intervention that organizers believed was effective despite expert criticism), and screening of the most traumatized in a group format. Afterward, the psychosocial support headquarters began a professional group intervention for traumatized people; each screened-positive survivor attended 3 weekly sessions of group cognitive behavior therapy. Based on some evidence, these interventions were recognized as efficient for the prevention and decrease of symptoms and the frequency of posttraumatic stress disorder (PTSD).[25–29]

FIRST-YEAR SOCIOECONOMIC AND MENTAL HEALTH IMPACT

The residents of the earthquake-stricken city of Bam, like the survivors of other disasters around the world, after the acute phase of addressing basic needs experienced acute grief and stress reactions and temporary settlement and then faced new psychological problems as they engaged in new business-related, economic, and social issues in the longer term. New symptoms of psychological problems appeared.

Although the agricultural part of the Bam economy, which was dependent on date palms, was not significantly affected by the quake, Bam's subterranean canals, which were the water source for other forms of agriculture, were damaged. Additionally, many farmers died and many farmlands were left unattended. Arg-é Bam was destroyed completely, not only affecting lost tourism and the economy (see **Fig. 3**) but also having a significant negative impact on the identity of Bam citizens for whom it was a civic symbol. A large group of working class people, however, immigrated to Bam to find a job and make a living from the humanitarian and public projects related to recovery. Immigrants also helped in picking and packing the dates, which was of help to the people of Bam who had lost their family members. Still, Bam citizens were not happy about the presence of these immigrants and realistically considered them a threat to their future employment. For example, more than Bam's people, they took possession of most connexes to use them as stores (a *connex* is a 9–12 m squared temporary, prefabricated living space that has no toilet, bathroom, or kitchen facilities). The products, such as clothes, that they were selling were sometimes also counter to the culture of Bam. The final outcome was that the survivors' average income decreased by two-thirds compared with their income before the earthquake.[7]

Iran is a large country and consists of different ethnicities, languages, accents, and cultures; thus, there were significant cultural differences between immigrants from other cities and the people of Bam. Therefore, immigrants from elsewhere greatly affected the cultural fabric of Bam. Unemployment, economic problems, broken families, and immigration together fostered an increase in the number of drug dealers (especially minor drug dealers) and made illicit drugs easily accessible.[24] The people of Bam believed the immigrants responsible for these social dilemmas in Bam (such as addiction, aggression, theft, and other crimes).[30]

After 8 months after the earthquake, an epidemiologic survey of the status of perceived social support in 786 Bam survivors was performed on survivors ages 15 and over,[21] among the respondents, 73.5% described their families' support as moderate to excellent, but 70.2% were not satisfied with their friends' support. Only 51.7% were covered by a health insurance system, although 73.7% of these people covered by the health insurance did not have any idea of the percentage of the fees paid by the insurance system. Approximately 78.9% were not covered by any social insurance system, but 92.8% of the insured were moderately to well satisfied with their insurance. More than 80% believed that performance of the media was moderate or excellent. Some complained about received aid and poor access to aid, and, more importantly, 71.3% of the respondents reported that social justice was poor. Approximately 12.6% of survivors were not satisfied with religious supports.

The grief process in a significant number of citizens was not normal. According to a study, 76% of survivors could not deal with the death of their relatives[31] and were still in deep grief months after the disaster. This occurred more commonly among women, illiterate people, and those who had experienced more severe psychological distress. Two different studies, both done during the first months after the quake, reported a 58% prevalence rate for severe psychological problems in Bam earthquake survivors above 15 years of age according to the 12-item General Health Questionnaire. These studies showed that these problems were more significant in women, illiterates, and unemployed and lonely people.[32,33]

Many of the survivors suffered from PTSD. According to the first study done after the quake based on *Diagnostic and Statistical Manual of Mental Disorders* (Fourth Edition) criteria, approximately 81% of survivors had PSTD.[34] Another study, done approximately 8 months after the earthquake, showed that the lifetime prevalence of this disorder in people more than age 15 years was 59.1% whereas its current prevalence at the time of study was 51.9%.[7] Although Iran was involved in an unwanted 8-year war with Iraq before the earthquake and people suffered the consequences, 97.1% of survivors believed that the Bam earthquake and its immediate consequences were responsible for their PSTD. In a study 8 months after the earthquake, 98.1% of those suffering from PSTD associated with the event still had the symptoms,[7] and there was a risk of them becoming chronic. This prevalence was even much higher than the rate reported in earthquakes in other parts of the world.[35–39] This may be because of the magnitude of Bam's destruction as well as the sensitivity of the surveying method in diagnosing the disorder.[7] Another important finding was that 20.2% of the population (half of those without this disorder) suffered from partial PTSD.[7] In this study, like Stein and colleagues',[40] each individual who had only 1 criterion of the B, C, and D criteria along with other criteria of PTSD was considered a partial PTSD patient. Although the dysfunction of partial PTSD patients could be due to a psychiatric comorbidity,[41] it indicates that detecting just PTSD in disaster survivors is not sufficient for screening cases in need of intervention, and further screening tests and interventions are recommended. Thus, patients have to be evaluated based on the presence of symptoms, not just a diagnosis.[42,43] Another important point is that 87.2% of survivors believed that the worst trauma was witnessing others' injuries or death and not the quake itself. This finding, that PTSD was more prevalent in vicarious trauma, has been discussed in other studies as well.[44] Therefore, when providing services to disaster survivors, it is necessary to take care of those who experienced the trauma indirectly at least as much as the ones who remained under the rubble.

Schools resumed their activity in the connexes after a month, and approximately 80% of the students enrolled. But due to decreased motivation and despair, only a small group decided to continue studying.[12] The students had lost many friends and classmates because of death or immigration, and the new classmates, who were the children of the immigrants, had not experienced the earthquake and even would pretend to have suffered through this experience. For months, students were complaining about lacking concentration to do their homework.[12] According to a study 4 months after the earthquake, 51.6% of the students younger than 15 years and 36.3% of those older than 15 years who had moved to Kerman after the quake were suffering from PTSD. Factors like female gender, young age, and being detached from the family after the trauma played a significant role in being affected by this disorder.[45] Although this prevalence rate (36.3%) was significant, it was much lower than the 51.9% prevalence rate among those who stayed in Bam.[7]

The Bam earthquake, like many other disasters in the world,[23,46] had an impact on substance abuse. It seemed that from the first days after the quake, use of illicit drugs (especially opium, which was the traditional one) increased. One study, done 2 months after the earthquake, showed that 8.3% of adults had an opioid addiction history before the incident whereas 9.9% became addicted after the quake.[20] After 8 months, 20.5% of men and 2.3% of women were using at least 1 illegal drug[47] and 25.1% of men and 4.1% of women reported using opium 8 months after the quake, whereas this rate was 17.4% in men and 3% in women 1 month before the earthquake. In general, 18.2% of men and 2.3% of women reported an increase in consumption of opioids after the incident.[47] Change in alcohol consumption by men before and after the quake was insignificant. These statistics are similar to those obtained from other parts of the world, where an increase in alcohol consumption was reported after disasters, but religious beliefs and Islamic restrictions precluded this in Bam (in Iran, alcohol is religiously prohibited whereas drugs, such as opiates and stimulants, are only illegal).[23,46] A year after the earthquake, all reports were indicative of a high consumption of opioid drugs in the villages surrounding Bam and its increased rate after the quake.[30] Substance abuse increased among children and women; 30% to 40% of all people referred to addiction rehabilitation centers had started using illicit drugs after the quake.[30] Addiction to heroin, which was not common before the incident, increased as well. Physicians estimated the prevalence of heroin consumption among those referred to substance abuse clinics to be 5% to 15%.[30] Because of the higher death toll in intravenous drug users as a result of their poor health and fragile living conditions during the first months after the quake, the prevalence of injection drug use decreased, but, during the first year after the quake, the group consumption of illicit drugs and incidence of high-risk behaviors gradually increased.[30]

During the first year after the earthquake, the psychosocial support headquarters continued its efforts to provide psychosocial interventions. For example, after a year, approximately 430 psychologists and psychiatrists, 105 school counselors, 1380 teachers, and hundreds of other health workers were trained in psychosocial support techniques by the Ministry of Health, and total coverage (more than 84,000 survivors in 21,000 tents, who identified as screen positive during the first session, received assistance) of mental health interventions was achieved. There were also activities in schools, recreation centers for children, public meetings, and activities aimed at special groups. Group play therapy was effective in reducing posttraumatic symptoms in preschool-aged children.[48] Trauma counseling of teachers was done directly by Ministry of Health professionals or indirectly through trained school counselors. The community-based psychosocial interventions were initiated with the help of trained local health volunteers. Public meetings with the people led by the psychosocial teams were held to help empower the people to rebuild their lives. A total of 135 health volunteers were trained by intervention teams in 4 workshops. They were laypeople and most of them were ordinary housewives. They were trained how to build local networks and do problem finding and problem solving with the people themselves. Steps were also taken to assist the survivors overcome their familial, occupational, and economic problems. A mobile library was developed by the social working team and distributed by health volunteers.

LONG-TERM SOCIOECONOMIC AND MENTAL HEALTH IMPACT

There is a lack of evidence-based data on the course of survivors during the years after the Bam earthquake, suggesting that Bam disaster survivors, despite their great loss, may have been ignored by the scientific associations and policy makers. To find more information, the authors conducted a qualitative study. The following represents findings from individual deep interviews with key informants and mental health professionals as well as focus group discussions with Bam residents. Based on the findings, the health system of the region (led by Kerman Medical University) continued to provide services to Bam survivors for a year, but the services were not consistent after the first year.

The impacts of Bam earthquake did not appreciably disappear, even after a long time, but instead their form changed. The long-term effects underscored how disasters can significantly change the socioeconomic status of survivors. For example, according to Iran civil law, in cases of death of an individual, the heirs are the children and spouse; if a deceased individual does not have a spouse or children, then the heirs are the siblings; if there are no siblings, the siblings' children are the heirs. Because in the Bam earthquake the death toll was enormous, the majority of survivors lost many relatives and many of them received inheritances. Therefore, after the earthquake and probate, the poor suddenly became wealthier and their socioeconomic status improved. Meanwhile, there were also those from the higher class who not only did not inherit much but also lost all of their assets at once and dropped to a lower class.

An important factor in influencing the postdisaster socioeconomic status of survivors was their type of business. Government employees enjoyed job stability more than other workers. Businessmen and shopkeepers did not and thus incurred more loss than others. This group of workers lost their business location, their goods were damaged or stolen, and the connexes given to them as a business place were reallotted to the immigrants.

Another factor responsible for changes in the socioeconomics of Bam was the services provided by governmental organizations. With the onset of reconstruction of the city, those who were not previously qualified for a job found new job opportunities. Additionally, those who were poor before the quake started to take advantage of the public support services and, for example, were given housing, leading to significant improvement in their quality of life. These sudden changes had some positive outcomes, including a decrease in the number of beggars. It, however, changed public expectations, destabilized social relations, and, consequently, caused great stress, especially in those who dropped to a lower socioeconomic level.

The majority of those who had immigrated to Bam in the first days after the earthquake now resided there. Meanwhile, immigration from nearby villages affected the social relations in their original villages that were not hit by the earthquake. Given the chaotic condition of the city, most Bam residents who could afford to start a new life outside Bam immigrated to nearby cities in the first months after the earthquake. Consequently, after a few years, the number of skilled teachers decreased in Bam, and they were replaced by less experienced ones. This population turnover had an impact on the socioeconomic fabric of Bam and precipitated a drop in the overall socioeconomic status of the city.

The Iranian government assumed the lead in providing significant financial assistance to the people of Bam from the first days after the quake. At the beginning, aid was provided in small amounts, and people spent it on their daily needs. After a few months, however, the government paid 10,000,000 rials per deceased to a family. At that time, with the city completely ruined and people not having a roof over their heads (**Fig. 5**), this action was encouraging and instilled hope for peoples' lives. Because many people had no comparable plan for the future and lacked motivation to work, however, they spent their money on motorcycles or cars—this was true even for those who did not have such vehicles prior to the quake. This resulted in heavy traffic in Bam, risky driving, and increased rates of death and injuries due to car accidents. People believed these dangerous behaviors were because of despair about the future and lack of fear of death, but absence of a driving culture and societal distress may also be responsible.

Presence of immigrants from other cities and nearby villages and close interaction between the survivors and humanitarian organizations resulted in the formation of a newly mixed culture. This phenomenon jeopardized the traditional culture of Bam society that previously was a protective factor against social conflicts. As immigrants

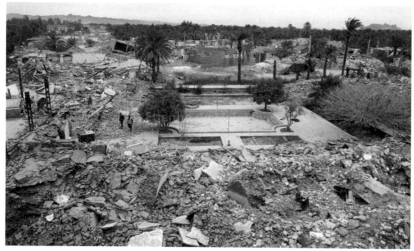

Fig. 5. Bam after earthquake.

started to interact with Bam citizens socially and occupationally, problems frequently arose due to cultural differences. For example, the marriages that occurred between immigrants and Bam people were mostly unsuccessful and resulted in divorce.

Most of the international nongovernmental organizations (NGOs) that came to Bam initially stayed for a long time. Because of the October 2005 Pakistan earthquake, however, most of these NGOs left Bam for Pakistan, because the situation in Bam had become relatively stable. After that, some citizens who were influenced by a culture of charity cultivated by and established local NGOs, including those for supporting orphaned children and providing nursing and shelter for them. Although these cultural changes were advantageous in some ways, in most cases, facing the new culture was stressful for Bam citizens and resulted in social mismatch, disintegration of traditional social relations, and, paradoxically, a decreased sense of social support. The impact of imported cultures was more prominent in women. Women's appearance and dressing styles gradually changed. This change of appearance in women sensitized the patriarchal culture of Bam and caused jealousy, bigotry, and family conflicts, which, in some cases led to broken families. Unfortunately, no specific investigation has been done on this subject.

Reconstruction of houses was started from the first months after the earthquake; involving people in the reconstruction process brought a sense of usefulness and a promising future, which had positive effects on people's mental health. The people of Bam were generally satisfied with governmental aid, although they thought public assistances were more than the governmental ones. Some loans were also given for purposes of reconstruction, but, for most people, especially those without a consistent income, paying back the loans was problematic. The government oversaw the reconstruction process, and paid part of the rebuilding expenses according to the rules and regulations. People could reconstruct their houses under the supervision of engineers approved by the government. As a result, those who used to have large houses now had to build 70-m to a 100-m houses, causing a change in their lifestyle. Reconstruction brought many contractors from other cities to Bam, but some reconstruction companies and the corrupted bureaucracy in which they operated were disappointing. Some of the stricken people of Bam found their new houses incompatible with their actual needs and number of their family members compared with their previous houses. With the onset of reconstruction in Bam, the construction-related businesses, including block factories, mosaic stores, and construction material shops, were considered positive. Those who were professionally involved in reconstruction appreciated, however, that this would not last forever and that the reconstruction process would soon decelerate. Therefore, although this process brought economic development, it did not create any sustained sense of job security or of a promising future.

One of the foremost issues after the quake was the quality of education. The school buildings were renovated and remodeled, which had a positive effect on students. Most students had psychological issues, however, due to the death or immigration of loved ones, classmates, and teachers. Also, the presence of immigrant students who were complete strangers to them further added to the problem. Thus, overall, quality of education and students' grades dropped.

The presence of various psychological disorders among Bam citizens also posed a significant problem for a long time after the quake. Generally, mental health services were promoted in the postdisaster phase compared with the predisaster phase; however, the majority of people and key informants believed that psychosocial support services in the first year were intensive, but, after that, the health system left people without adequate services. The drop in the quality of life of Bam's people in all aspects, including physical health, psychological status, social relations, and environment, was clear. This decrease in quality of life was more significant in the elderly, women, those who lived alone, those who sustained more significant injury, residents of the suburbs, and those who were more dependent on others for living.[49] For instance, approximately 300 to 400 people had spinal cord injury. As discussed in other studies,[50,51] paralysis and physical illnesses are among the risk factors for decreased quality of life of survivors.[49,52] Meanwhile, the greater the prevalence of psychological problems due to the quake, the lower the survivors' quality of life.[53,54]

The grief recovery process was a significant clinical issue observed in traumatized Bam earthquake survivors for those who had had lost relatives as well as social and financial assets. The grief process in such people was severe and became chronic in many cases, lasting for several years and sometimes mistakenly diagnosed as major depressive disorder. Some people suffering from complicated grief grappled with thoughts of suicide. A major difference between this long-term grief and depressive disorders seems that anhedonia was not a common symptom of the former. The main symptom of prolonged grief was agitation and, less commonly, helplessness and worthlessness. Most importantly, response to psychotropic medications was limited.

Mental health experts believed that one of the important issues was a higher prevalence of clinical depression in the population during the years after the quake, mostly in the form of psychomotor agitation and not retarded depression. Agitation seems to have contributed to aggression and violence. According to the Kerman University of Medical Sciences annual report, suicide attempts and completed suicide decreased in the city; the year after the quake completed suicide was 5.2 per 100,000 compared with 9 per 100,000 before the quake (Kerman University of Medical Sciences, unpublished data, 2005). Some clinicians reported that most of these completed suicides were attempted by addicted people. The rate of suicide was 6 per 100,000 in 2011 (Kerman University of Medical Sciences, unpublished data, 2012).

A psychiatrist residing in Bam observed that after 2 years, approximately 20% to 30% of the people suffering from PTSD still had their disorder. He considered this rate higher than the pre-earthquake prevalence rate in the city but did not have a precise prevalence rate (Mohsen Hafezi, MD, Bam, Iran, personal communication, October 2012).

The most common experienced symptoms in PTSD sufferers involved hypervigilance. This disorder caused a severe reduction in people's functioning. Students diagnosed with PTSD experienced academic failure and sometimes even dropped out.

As expected from the course of substance dependence, it did not decrease to its previous rate after increasing after the disaster. The chronicity of PTSD symptoms after the traumatic event seems to be responsible for one-fifth of illicit drug use that started after the quake. Unfortunately, injection drug use, which had decreased during the first months after the quake, increased even more than before, and intravenous users started to show more risky behaviors, such as unprotected sex and violence. Considering the changed pattern of illicit drug use from opiates to stimulants in the entire country, traditional opium was replaced by amphetamine-type drugs in Bam. A separate study is required to specifically evaluate and focus on the difference between this change throughout the country and in the city of Bam and its correlation with the earthquake. Due to the higher demand for illicit drugs and increased rate of addiction and unemployment, drug trafficking increased during the years after the quake.

IMPLICATIONS FOR MENTAL HEALTH WORKERS IN FUTURE DISASTERS

The Bam earthquake caused a range of negative outcomes. It significantly changed the public culture, increased ethical problems, disturbed socioeconomic relations and balance, and increased the prevalence of psychiatric disorders. This earthquake had significant impacts, far more than the destruction of buildings and the city, and left extensive long-term effects on different aspects of people's lives, which may last for decades.

In spite of every second of sorrow, the Bam earthquake and the recovery efforts that followed hold valuable lessons for all of society, policy makers in the health system, and health specialists and health care workers in this field.

Nationwide Capacity Building to Deliver Psychosocial Services

Considering the social and mental damage caused by most disasters, it is necessary to increase national capacity for the delivery of psychosocial services far more than was the case in the Bam earthquake. Approximately 20% of Bam's health care workers who were not specifically in charge of providing mental health services died during the incident, which caused a significant shortage of trained human resources. Surviving health care workers are not capable of providing services for a long time due to the physical and psychological toll of this work, especially when they personally experienced the trauma.

Employment of Different Levels of Psychological Services

Reports regarding the delivery of social and psychological supports in Bam show that psychological services were widely provided for the survivors, especially during the first year. But, to the best of the authors' knowledge, no study has evaluated the long-term effectiveness of the postearthquake mental health interventions supported by the Ministry of Health. The large number of people in need necessitated that psychological services were short term and limited to the common and the predetermined service package of screening followed by 3 group psychotherapy sessions. Mahmoudi-Gharaei and colleagues[55] reported that interventions were helpful but as effective as encouraging kids to play soccer. Therefore, a more systematic and precise plan should be implemented for delivering psychological services, like crisis counseling[56] or emotion regulation,[57] in cases resistant to primary interventions. Thus, there should be records for delivering more comprehensive services during the second 6 months after the earthquake.

Providing Resources Necessary for the Regional Consistency of Service Delivery with the Help of Specialized Local Forces

In the long-term aftermath of the Bam earthquake, responsibility for health and mental health service delivery fell to the health system of the region and specialized local staff. In retrospect, the results of this strategy in Bam shows that assigning responsibility for health/mental health service delivery to local agencies, without manpower capacity building and allocation of necessary budgets, is not enough. Additionally, it seems that designing a plan for controlling quality and quantity of services is a necessity for effectively implementing such a comprehensive strategy.

Reinforcing Social Supports and Psychological Interventions

The profound impact of proper social supports, including government assistance and helping people organize self-help groups, especially survivors' perception of these supports, reinforces the effect of psychological interventions on survivors[35,58] and can even decrease the destructive effects of a traumatic event.[39,59,60] Unfortunately, in many developing countries, the social support networks are not consistent or strong enough, and people with special needs are not given enough attention and are marginalized.[61] Naturally, this deficiency becomes more prominent in times of disaster, when people are desperately in need of even more social supports. Bam survivors' points of view revealed that the weakness of social support networks decreased the effectiveness of psychological interventions.

It seems that the social support structure must be designed according to a society's existing structures and capacities as well as types of relations. Additionally, supports, especially financial aid, should be delivered at the right time and according to a plan. For instance, most survivors in Bam thought their major social support source was their relatives.[21] Therefore, social support services would be provided better through relatives. This is not a general rule, however, and may change in different cultures. In some societies, this support may be provided through friends or other social resources, including humanitarian organizations.

Integration of Pharmaceutical or Nonpharmaceutical Therapy in Survivors

Some studies have suggested that proper and short-term prescription of psychotropic medications during a disaster would prevent psychological disorders and could effectively treat patients.[62–64] For instance, Katz and colleagues[63] showed that psychotropic drugs were prescribed for 47% of September 11th survivors who were mostly diagnosed with psychological disorders. This finding highlights the important role of psychiatrists compared with other health care workers.[65] Review of the activities of the socioeconomic support committee in Bam revealed that the general policy supported only nonpharmaceutical interventions and only a minority were referred by mobile teams to outpatient psychiatric clinics for medication. Despite the effectiveness of nonpharmaceutical interventions reported in the Bam earthquake[25,28,29,48] and other similar events,[35] the potential efficacy of pharmaceutical therapies emphasizes the point that more widespread use of these therapies may significantly improve effectiveness of provided services.

Delivery of Services by Specialists Who are Acquainted with the Stricken Area in Term of Cultural and Lingual Characteristics

One priority of the social and psychological support committee in Bam was to use local, or at least Kermani, psychologists. Due to some restrictions, however, some involved psychologists were from other provinces. This caused some problems: first, many of the survivors believed that these psychologists had not experienced the trauma and, therefore, could not understand their problems; second, cultural difference was an excuse for the survivors not to accept them.

Delivery of Psychological Services by Mobile Teams

Experience shows that delivery of social and psychological supports through structured systems based at health centers, especially during the first days and months after the quake, was not enough in satisfying the needs. Therefore, an approach based on psychological service delivery through outreach teams is vital. Likewise, working in, at times, an informal manner and relying on laypersons who have participated in basic mental health training courses may also be effective.

ACKNOWLEDGMENTS

The authors would like to thank Drs Javad Mahmoudi Gharaei, Zohreh Ghafari, Mohsen Hafezi, and Khashayar Khamisizadeh; Ms ZeinabeSarhadi; Nahid Kaviani; and Mr Mohammad Danesh Jahangard, whose kind cooperation made this research possible.

REFERENCES

1. Cohen J, Uphoff N. Rural development participation: concepts and measures for project design, implementation and evaluation. Ithaca (NY): 2003. Available at: http://www.popline.org/node/499235. Accessed June 23, 2013.
2. Delaney P. Humanitarianism and participation: moving beyond DO NO Harm in disaster mitigation and Response. In: Ottawa, Canada: A Call to Action, Participatory Development Forum; 2003.
3. Ebrahimpour M. Social outcomes of Bam earthquake in traumatized villages. J Rural Dev Stud 2009;11:175.
4. Kerman Province, Wikipedia, the free encyclopedia, in, 2012, Vol 20/11/2012. Available at: http://en.wikipedia.org/wiki/Kerman_Province. Accessed June 23, 2013.
5. Arman-Shahr Engineering Consulting Company. In: Report on comprehensive plan of Bam City (12 volumes). Kerman Province Press; 2010.
6. Management and Planning Organization. Statistical yearbook of Kerman province. In: Tehran (Iran): Kerman Province Press; 2002.
7. Farhoudian A, Sharifi V, Rahmi Movaghar A, et al. The prevalence of posttraumatic stress disorder and its symptoms among Bam earthquake survivors. Advances Cognitive Science 2006;8:58.
8. Noorbala AA, Yazdi SA. Mental health survey of the adult population in Iran. Br J Psychiatry 2004;184:70.
9. Chen KT, Chen WJ, Malilay J, et al. The public health response to the Chi-Chi earthquake in Taiwan, 1999. Public Health Rep 2003;118:493.
10. Moszynski P. Cold is the main health threat after the Bam earthquake. BMJ 2004; 328:66.
11. Yasamy M, Farajpour M, Gudarzi S, et al. First seven months of psychosocial intervention in Bam. Department of mental health, Ministry of Health and Medical Education; 2004.
12. EERI Special Earthquake Report, Learning from Earthquakes: Social and Public Policy Issues following the Bam, Iran, Earthquake, in, 2004. Available at: https://www.eeri.org/lfe/pdf/Iran_Bam_Insert2_Aug04.pdf. Accessed June 23, 2013.

13. Rahimi Movaghar A, Farhoudian A, Rad Goodarzi R, et al. A survey on changes in opioid use and risk factors in the survivors eight months after Bam earthquake. Tehran University Medical Journal 2006;64(6):77–94.
14. Mohamadi L, Mohamadkhani P, Dolatshahi B, et al. Posttraumatic stress disorder symptoms and their comorbidity with other disorders in eleven to sixteen years old adolescents in the city of Bam. Iranian Journal Psychiatry Clinical Psychology 2010;16:187.
15. Jazayeri A, Ebrahimi M. Disaster management plan of the Islamic Republic of Iran, in the Second International Conference on Seismology and Earthquake Engineering. Tehran (Iran): 1995.
16. Akbari ME, Farshad AA, Asadi-Lari M. The devastation of Bam: an overview of health issues 1 month after the earthquake. Public Health 2004;118:403.
17. Bolhari J, Chime N. Mental health intervention in Bam earthquake crisis: a qualitative Study. Tehran University Medical Journal 2007;65:7.
18. Rad Goodarzi R, Rahimi Movaghar A, Sahimi Izadian E, et al. The approach of health system in dealing with opioid withdrawal symptoms in Bam earthquake victims during the first two weeks after the disaster. J Sch Publ Health Inst Publ Health Res 2005;3:1.
19. Tavakoli H, Farajzadeh D. Jonaidi Jafari N: the study of providing, preservation and distribution of foodstuffs in Bam earthquake. Journal Military Medicine 2008;10:11.
20. Bayanzadeh A, Eslami YA, Sam Aram EA, et al. An investigation about the living conditions of Bam earthquake survivals. Soc Welfare 2004;3:113.
21. Farhoudian A, Rahimi Movaghar A, Rad Goodarzi R, et al. Social support among Bam earthquake survivors. University of Social Welfare and Rehabilitation Science. Final Report, 2005.
22. Sahimi Izadian E, Rahimi Movaghar A, Rad Goodarzi R, et al. Withdrawal symptoms in drug dependents in Bam during the first two weeks after the earthquake. Social Welfare 2004;3:133.
23. Vlahov D, Galea S, Ahern J, et al. Sustained Increased Consumption of Cigarettes, Alcohol, and Marijuana among Manhattan Residents After September11, 2001. Am J Public Health 2004;94:253.
24. Rad Goodarzi R, Rahimi Movaghar A, Farhoudian A, et al. A qualitative study of changes in supplying of illicit drugs in Bam during the first year after the earthquake. Social Welfare 2006;5:163.
25. Fakour Y, Mahmoudi-gharaei J, Mohammadi MR, et al. The effect of supportive and cognitive behavioral group therapy on Bam earthquake survivors with Post Traumatic Stress Disorder. Hakim Research Journal 2006;9:63.
26. Fakour Y, Mohammadi MR, Mahmoudi-Gharaei J, et al. The effect of psychosocial debriefing and behavioral grop interventions on symptoms of posttraumatic stress disorder in survivors of Bam earthquake. Advance Cognitive Science 2006;6:3.
27. Fan F, Zhang Y, Yang Y, et al. Symptoms of posttraumatic stress disorder, depression, and anxiety among adolescents following the 2008 Wenchuan earthquake in China. J Trauma Stress 2011;14.
28. Mahmoudi-Gharaei J, Mohammadi MR, Bina M, et al. Behavioral group therapy effect on Bam earthquake related PTSD symptoms in children: a randomized clinical trial. Iran J Pediatr 2006;16:25.
29. Shooshtary MH, Panaghi L, Moghadam JA. Outcome of cognitive behavioral therapy in adolescents after natural disaster. J Adolesc Health 2008;42:466.

30. Farhoudian A, Rahimi Movaghar A, Rad Goodarzi R, et al. Changes in the use of opioid drugs and available interventions in Bam during the First Year after the Earthquake. Hakim 2006;9:52.
31. Ghaffari-Nejad A, Ahmadi-Mousavi M, Gandomkar M, et al. The prevalence of complicated grief among Bam earthquaqe survivors in Iran. Arch Iran Med 2007;10:525.
32. Hagh-Shenas H, Goodarzi MA, Dehbozorgi G, et al. Psychological consequences of the Bam earthquake on professional and nonprofessional helpers. J Trauma Stress 2005;18:477.
33. Montazeri A, Baradaran H, Omidvari S, et al. Psychological distress among Bam earthquake survivors in Iran: a population-based study. BMC Public Health 2005;11:54.
34. Hagh-Shenas H, Goodarzi MA, Farajpoor M, et al. Post-traumatic stress disorder among survivors of Bam earthquake 40 days after the event. East Mediterr Health J 2006;12:118.
35. Kar N. Psychological impact of disasters on children: review of assessment and interventions. World J Pediatr 2009;5:5–11.
36. Kiliç C, Ulusoy M. Psychological effects of the November 1999 earthquake in Turkey: an epidemiological study. Acta Psychiatr Scand 2003;108:2328.
37. Kuo C-J, Tang H-S, Tsay C-J, et al. Prevalence of Psychiatric Disorders among bereaved survivors of a disastrous earthquake in Taiwan. Psychiatr Serv 2003; 54:249–51.
38. Priebe S, Grappasonni I, Mari M, et al. Posttraumatic stress disorder six months after an earthquake: findings from a community sample in a rural region in Italy. Soc Psychiatry Psychiatr Epidemiol 2009;44:393.
39. Wang X, Gao L, Shinfuku N, et al. Longitudinal study of earthquake-related PTSD in a randomly Selected community sample in North China. Am J Psychiatry 2000;157:1260.
40. Stein MB, Walker JR, Hazen AL, et al. Full and partial posttraumatic stress disorder: findings from a community survey. Am J Psychiatry 1997;154:1114.
41. Shiner B, Bateman D, Young-Xu Y, et al. Comparing the stability of diagnosis in full vs. partial posttraumatic stress disorder. J Nerv Ment Dis 2012;200:520.
42. Gudmundsdottir B, Beck JG. Understanding the pattern of PTSD symptomatology: a comparison of between versus within-group approaches. Behav Res Ther 2004;42:1367.
43. Pietrzak RH, Schechter CB, Bromet EJ, et al. The burden of full and subsyndromal posttraumatic stress disorder among police involved in the World Trade Center rescue and recovery effort. J Psychiatr Res 2012;46:835–42.
44. Saxon AJ, Davis TM, Sloan KL, et al. Trauma, symptoms of posttraumatic stress disorder, and associated problems among incarcerated veterans. Psychiatr Serv 2001;52:959.
45. Parvaresh N, Bahramnezhad A. Post-traumatic stress disorder in bam-survived students who immigrated to Kerman, four months after the earthquake. Arch Iran Med 2009;12:244.
46. Pfefferbaum B, Vinekar SS, Trautman RP, et al. The Effect of loss and trauma on substance use behavior in individuals seeking support services after the 1995 Oklahoma city bombing. Ann Clin Psychiatry 2002;14:89.
47. Rahimi Movaghar A, Farhoudian A, Rad Goodarzi R, et al. A survey on changes in opioid use and risk factors in the survivors eight months after Bam earthquake. Tehran University Medical Journal 2006;64:77.

48. Mahmoudi-Gharaei J, Bina M, Yasami MT, et al. Group play therapy effect on Bam earthquake related emotional and behavioral symptoms in preschool children: a before-after trial. Iran J Pediatr 2006;16:137.

49. Ardalan A, Mazaheri M, Vanrooyen M, et al. Post-disaster quality of life among older survivors five years after the Bam earthquake: implications for recovery policy. Ageing Soc 2011;31:179.

50. Ceyhan E, Ceyhan AA. Earthquake survivors' quality of life and academic achievement six years after the earthquakes in Marmara, Turkey. Disasters 2007;31:516.

51. Wu HC, Chou P, Chou FH, et al. Survey of quality of life and related risk factors for a Taiwanese village population 3 years post-earthquake. Aust N Z J Psychiatry 2006;40:335.

52. Ardalan A, Mazaheri M, Mowafi H, et al. Impact of the 26 December 2003 Bam Earthquake on activities of daily living and instrumental activities of daily living of older people. Prehospital Disaster Med 2011;26:99.

53. Chou FHC, Chou P, Lin C, et al. The relationship between quality of life and psychiatric impairment for a Taiwanese community post-earthquake. Qual Life Res 2004;13:1089.

54. Tsai KY, Chou P, Chou FH, et al. Three-year follow-up study of the relationship between posttraumatic stress symptoms and quality of life among earthquake survivors in Yu-Chi, Taiwan. J Psychiatr Res 2007;41:90.

55. Mahmoudi-Gharaei J, Mohammadi MR, Yasami MT, et al. Group cognitive-behavior therapy and supportive art and sport interventions on Bam earthquake related post traumatic stress symptoms in children: a field trial. Iranian Journal Psychiatry Clinical Psychology 2009;4:85.

56. Rosen CS, Greene CJ, Young HE, et al. Tailoring disaster mental health services to diverse needs: an analysis of 36 crisis counseling projects. Health Soc Work 2010;35:211.

57. Cameron CD, Payne BK. Escaping affect: how motivated emotion regulation creates insensitivity to mass suffering. J Pers Soc Psychol 2011;100:1.

58. Joseph S, Andrews B, Williams R, et al. Crisis support and psychiatric symptomatology in adult survivors of the Jupiter cruise ship disaster. Br J Clin Psychol 1992;31:63.

59. Cerdá M, Paczkowski M, Galea S, et al. Psychopathology in the aftermath of the Haiti earthquake: a population-based study of posttraumatic stress disorder and major depression. Depress Anxiety 2013;30(5):413–24.

60. Zhang Z, Wang W, Shi Z, et al. Mental health problems among the survivors in the hard-hit areas of the Yushu earthquake. PLoS One 2012;7:46449.

61. Kailes JI, Enders A. Moving beyond "special needs": a function based framework for emergency management and planning. J Disabil Pol Stud 2007;17:230.

62. Blaha J, Svobodova K, Kapounkova Z. Therapeutical aspects of using citalopram in burns. Acta Chir Plast 1999;41:25.

63. Katz CL, Pellegrino L, Pandya A, et al. Research on psychiatric outcomes and interventions subsequent to disasters: a review of the literature. Psychiatry Res 2002;110:201.

64. Robert R, Meyer WJ, Villarreal C, et al. An approach to the timely treatment of acute stress disorder. J Burn Care Rehabil 1999;20:250.

65. Pandya A, Katz CL, Smith R, et al. Services provided by volunteer psychiatrists after 9/11 at the New York City family assistance center: September 12-November 20, 2001. J Psychiatr Pract 2010;16:193.

Holistic Approach to Community in Crisis

Sandip Shah, MD

KEYWORDS

- Earthquake • Mental health • Posttraumatic stress disorder • Volunteers

KEY POINTS

- After a devastating event, instead of waiting for the approval by authorities, treatment should be started as early as possible to increase the possibility for positive outcomes and shorten the transition period to recovery.
- For better acceptance and results, one should integrate mental health approaches into local traditions and customs.
- Mental health efforts should first reach the rural areas and those without television coverage.
- The period of transition from relief to recovery is the most critical for mental health.

BACKGROUND

The Kachchh district in Gujarat, with an area of 45,652 km², is the largest district in India (**Fig. 1**).[1,2] The administrative headquarters is in Bhuj, which is geographically in the center of the district. Other main towns are Gandhidham, Rapar, Nakhatrana, Anjar, Mandvi, Madhapar, and Mundra. Kachchh has 966 villages (**Fig. 2**). According to the 2001 census, Kutch district had a population of 1,583,225. According to the 2011 census, this grew to 2,090,313, indicating a population growth rate of 32.03% over the decade 2001 to 2011. Kutch is a growing economic and industrial hub in one of India's fastest growing states, Gujarat. Its location on the far western edge of India has resulted in the commissioning of 2 major ports Kandla and Mundra. In 2001 there was only 1 general hospital staffed with a single psychiatrist and 8 psychiatrists in private hospitals, reflecting the low awareness of mental health in Kachchh.

EARTHQUAKE DETAILS

The earthquake that hit Gujarat (see **Fig. 2**; **Fig. 3**) on the morning of January 26, 2001 left in its wake a trail of death and destruction, leaving a population of close to 500,000

Disclosure Statement: The Program was carried out by the NGO Indu Health Research Foundation (IHRF) and was supported by a grant from the Embassy of Netherlands, The ING Vyasya Bank. The Program Consultants are: (1) Dr Sandip Shah, (2) Dr Yoep Toebosch.
Department of Psychiatry, SBKS MI&RC, Sumandeep Vidyapeeth, Vadodara 391760, India
E-mail address: researchdirectorsvu@gmail.com

Psychiatr Clin N Am 36 (2013) 403–416
http://dx.doi.org/10.1016/j.psc.2013.05.010
0193-953X/13/$ – see front matter © 2013 Elsevier Inc. All rights reserved.

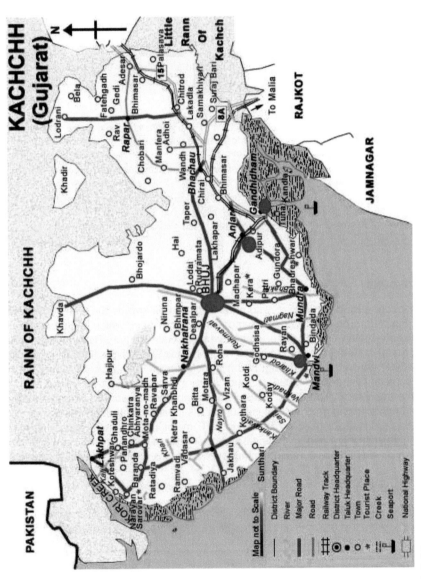

Fig. 1. Map of Kachchh.

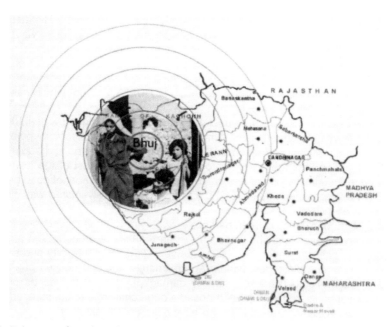

Fig. 2. Epicenter of earthquake.

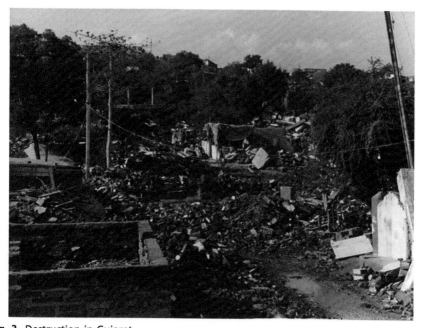

Fig. 3. Destruction in Gujarat.

homeless and almost 100,000 dead or seriously injured (unofficial estimates). The quake measured 6.9 on the Richter scale (7.7 as per the US Geological Survey), lasted for about 100 seconds, and shook the entire state of Gujarat. The epicenter of the earthquake lay 20 km to the north-east of Bhuj in the Kachchh district in Gujarat. About 16 million people in 21 districts out of 25 in Gujarat state were affected by the earthquake. The total loss was estimated at Rs. 700 crore (US$4.5 billion), which was about 15% of Gross Domestic Product in India.

In Kachchh several villages were decimated and literally flattened within 100 seconds. Massive infrastructure loss or damage to roads, bridges electricity poles, and telecommunication lines was recorded (**Fig. 4**). All civic amenities and supply lines ceased to function until they were restored after 48 hours. Most of the towns and villages had turned into heaps of rubble. The estimate of the number of dead beneath the rubble was more than 20,000, and the number of seriously injured was close to 200,000.

Although earthquakes have been part of the history of Kachchh (according to popular lore every 3 years Kachchh witnesses an earthquake, a drought. and a normal monsoon), the one on January 26, 2001 was very different in intensity and scale. It left behind near complete destruction (approximately 400,000 houses completely destroyed, about 700,000 houses partially damaged), claimed thousands of lives, and left thousands injured in Gujarat. It posed a huge challenge to the state administration to gear up to meet the rescue and relief needs of the situation.

The extent of damage in Kachchh during the 2001 earthquake is shown in **Table 1**.

Following the earthquake, several nongovernmental organizations (NGOs) within Gujarat came together under the banner of Citizens' Initiative, a broad platform of NGOs under the aegis of which several organizations became involved in relief operations.

The day after the earthquake, doctors of the Indian Medical Association branch of Vadodara and the Blood Bank of the Indu Health Research Foundation launched an initiative to provide medical aid to the survivors. After the initial rescue efforts, it became clear that this terrifying experience not only turned human lives upside

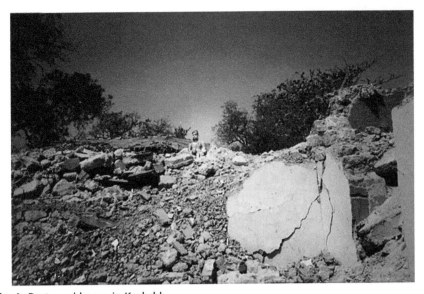

Fig. 4. Destroyed house in Kachchh.

Table 1
Extent of damage: loss of human lives, livestock, and property in Gujarat

No.	Indicators	Total Number in Gujarat	Total Number in Kachchh
1	Human deaths	19,904	18,315
2	Injured	166,061	136,048
3	Hospitalized patients	20,717	13,441
4	Animal deaths	21,258	20,100
5	Completely destroyed *Pucca* houses	171,622	106,986
6	Completely destroyed *Kuchha* houses	167,035	107,109
7	Partially destroyed *Pucca* houses	488,288	101,902

Pucca houses are houses built with cements and bricks. *Kuchha* houses are makeshift houses built using mud with a thatched roof.

Data from Gujarat: a devastating earthquake. Published by the Directorate of Information, Gujarat State.

down and left people with a sense of unpredictability and vulnerability, but also profoundly changed the manner in which they subsequently managed their emotions, their environment, and their very lives. To address these problems, a program was developed to help the survivors in the community to properly manage their earthquake-associated mental health problems and, hence, achieve a better physical and mental outcome.

PROGRESS AND METHODOLOGY

A practical manual for counselors on posttraumatic stress disorder (PTSD) was developed by Sandeep Shah (psychiatrist) and Joep Toebosch (specialist on PTSD-related problems), consisting of educational elements covering the following topics in brief:

- Causes and effects of PTSD
- The mechanism of relaxation
- The benefits of regular exercises
- Negative and irrational thinking and their effects on PTSD
- Yoga and progressive relaxation techniques

A total of 19,500 Gujarati survivors were approached, of whom 10,045 were screened, interviewed, and consequently rated on the prevalence of PTSD on a modified rating scale that specifically took into account the Indian extended family.[3] The scale consisted of 3 parts: A, B, and C. Parts A and B comprised 5 questions each related to problems of reliving the event, dreams, loss of interest, emotional blunting, sleep disturbance, irritability and concentration difficulties, anxiety, and startle. Part C comprised 5 questions related to mood: sadness, hopelessness, easy fatigability, loss of appetite, and indecisiveness. Items in parts A and B were rated as yes/no responses, and part C was rated on a Likert-type scale of 1 to 4. A total of 45 villages were covered under the PTSD project, beginning in April 2001.

The holistic community approach (**Fig. 5**) to the earthquake survivors is based on 4 kinds of "pillars." Counselor training involved learning relaxation techniques (group therapy and structured progressive muscular relaxation). The second pillar was Indian yoga, which was already deeply ingrained in the society and therefore easily adopted for mental health practice (**Fig. 6A–C**). The participants were taught

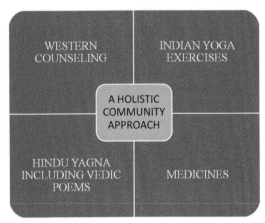

Fig. 5. The holistic community approach.

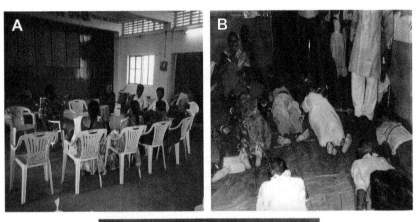

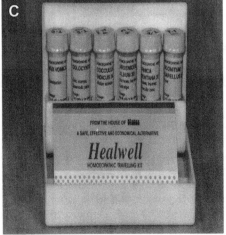

Fig. 6. (*A*) Meeting of group of 8 to 12 to share the experience of earthquake. (*B*) Relaxation and progressive muscular relaxation. (*C*) On prescription of psychiatrists, homeopathic, ayurvedic, and allopathic medicines are provided free.

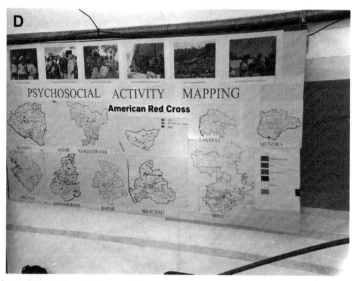

Fig. 6. (*D*) Psychosocial activity mapping.

preselected Yogasanas, which were targeted at progressive muscular relaxation using visual imagery and breathing techniques. Another important pillar and significantly "Indian" part of approach was the focus on spiritual rituals, which is typical of the people living in this geographic area. Rituals known as Yajnas, which appeared to bring spiritual relief to the survivors concerned, were organized at the end of a term in every village, when the project was finalized. (Here a term indicates the exit of counselors from the village at end of Yajna, which was typically 10 weeks' duration, as the medication was given for 8 weeks and 2 weeks were kept for data collection before and after.) The Yajna was organized in a traditional manner by the same expert from the Sanskrit Faculty of MS University, who with his team lit a fire in a brick enclave (*hawan kund*) in a specific manner using special ingredients and the chanting of mantras.

On average, at least 4 counselors were working on a permanent basis in any one village. These counselors were volunteers mostly from the faculty of Social Work or Psychology, and were at minimum graduates. All counselors underwent an orientation program on the subject of PTSD and what they would be required to do during their stay. Children were not included, as UNESCO was in charge of the child survivors. Counselors met the survivors daily as they were staying in the same village throughout the term, and held their meetings during the evening social gatherings of the village(s). All meetings included the Yogasanas, and were held once a week for 8 weeks.

Several psychiatrists (who were volunteer psychiatrists from in and around state of Gujarat, as the psychiatrists from the affected area were initially not in a fit state to offer their services) made their time and resources available for this project. The problems encountered by the survivors were brought to the attention of 1 of the 4 psychiatrists who visited every Sunday to observe the work done by the counselors and to prescribe the required medicines. Sertraline, a selective serotonin reuptake inhibitor, was administered for 8 weeks.[4,5] Sertraline was selected because the literature reviewed at that time mentioned sertraline, it was easily available in the area, and required once-daily dosing. The medicines were dispensed after the psychologists reported the survivor participant to have scored above the cutoff score on the administered scale and also consented to attend the Sunday clinic. The survivor was then seen by a psychiatrist and was dispensed medication for 8 weeks. The ayurvedic medicines were dispensed free of charge by an ayurvedic practitioner, mostly to address somatic complaints, and also were prescribed to those who demanded them.

UNICEF and the American Red Cross (see **Fig. 6D**) organized biweekly meetings by staff members in the city of Bhuj in the first few months as the government of Gujarat was not fully functioning, leaving a void on guidance on mental health issues.

RESULTS

During the project, a total of 19,500 Gujarati survivors were approached beginning in February 2001, of whom 10,045 were screened, interviewed, and consequently rated on the prevalence of PTSD on a modified rating scale for the diagnosis of PTSD (**Table 2**). Ultimately, 3315 survivors were subject to psychological intervention. All were survivors who scored above the cutoff level on the scale administered by the volunteers to rate PTSD (children were not included).

The most significant finding was longitudinal; that is, on examining the monthly distribution of survivors' ratings from February 2001 until December 2001, there is an 89.7% prevalence of PTSD symptoms in the first month, which gradually decreases monthly and stabilizes at around 21% in the 10th and 11th month.

Table 3 shows the rates of PTSD in the target population who underwent counselor-administered manualized psychological interventions from April to September 2001.

The data reflect the 3315 survivors rated from February to April and rerated after psychological intervention. There is a decrease in the percentage of PTSD-positive survivors from 89.7% in February to 18.6% in April, and a further decrease in the following months (**Fig. 7**).

Table 2
Overall PTSD prevalence (N = 10,045)

Parameter	Sex		PTSD Positive Total
	PTSD Positive Male (%)	PTSD Positive Female (%)	
Age (y)			
≤25	51.6	56.1	53.8
26–35	50.9	54.6	52.7
36–45	52.5	57.7	54.9
46–55	52.4	59.5	55.7
>55	47.1	56	51.4
Education			
Lower	50.7	56.5	53.4
Middle	53.4	56.6	54.9
Upper	54.6	49.5	52.5
Occupation			
Lower	50	56.6	53.3
Middle	56.3	55.3	56
Higher	54.3	51.1	53.5

Table 3
Rates of PTSD following the holistic intervention (N = 3315)

Month	Male			Female			Overall		
	<6	≥6	Total	<6	≥6	Total	<6	≥6	Total
April	37 (77.1%)	11 (22.9%)	48 (2.6%)	42 (85.7%)	7 (14.3%)	49 (3.4%)	79 (81.4%)	18 (18.6%)	97 (2.9%)
May	19 (82.6%)	4 (17.4%)	23 (1.2%)	35 (83.3%)	7 (16.7%)	42 (2.9%)	54 (83.1%)	11 (16.9%)	65 (2.0%)
June	182 (85.4%)	31 (14.6%)	213 (11.4%)	122 (77.7%)	35 (22.3%)	157 (10.9%)	304 (82.2%)	66 (17.8%)	370 (11.2%)
July	262 (83.2%)	53 (16.8%)	315 (16.9%)	130 (87.2%)	19 (12.8%)	149 (10.3%)	392 (84.5%)	72 (15.5%)	464 (14.0%)
August	314 (86.5%)	49 (13.5%)	363 (19.4%)	168 (87.5%)	24 (12.5%)	192 (13.3%)	482 (86.8%)	73 (13.2%)	555 (16.7%)
September	776 (85.6%)	131 (14.4%)	907 (48.5%)	696 (81.2%)	161 (18.8%)	857 (59.3%)	1472 (83.4%)	292 (16.6%)	1764 (53.2%)
Total	1590 (85.1%)	279 (14.9%)	1869 (100%)	1193 (82.5%)	253 (17.5%)	1446 (100%)	2783 (84.0%)	532 (16.0%)	3315 (100%)

PTSD-ABC (After Psychological Intervention)

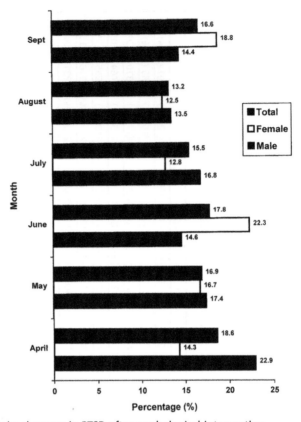

Fig. 7. Monthwise decrease in PTSD after psychological intervention.

Table 4 shows the response of the survivors to medication (sertraline) administered for 8 weeks; one can see a further decrease in the percentage of PTSD-positive survivors (ie, those who rated above the cutoff score) to 5.2%.

Fig. 8 shows a monthwise decrease in PTSD after medical treatment.

Fig. 9 shows the overall comparison of the effect of psychological intervention and medication in a group of survivors.

SUMMARY

This article addresses the postdisaster situation following the 2001 Gujarat earthquake and the effects of a holistic psychological intervention program on the mental health of the survivors. After such a devastating event, instead of waiting for the approval by authorities, treatment should be started as early as possible to increase the possibility for positive outcomes and shorten the transition period to recovery. The program screened for those at risk following earthquake and, with an early intervention in the form of medication, psychotherapy, relaxation exercises, and Yajna, an attempt was made to help people recognize their horror and loss in ways that would provide them with a significantly happier and less impaired future. Most importantly, the team observed that empathy, a healing touch, listening, and prayer, along with modern medical care, are what is needed by the disaster-affected population.

Table 4
Data of effect of medical treatment on PTSD-positive survivors after psychology intervention

Month	PTSD-ABC (After Medical Intervention)								
	Male			Female			Overall		
	<6	≥6	Total	<6	≥6	Total	<6	≥6	Total
June	45 (93.8%)	3 (6.3%)	48 (2.6%)	47 (95.9%)	2 (4.1%)	49 (3.4%)	92 (94.8%)	5 (5.2%)	97 (2.9%)
July	22 (95.7%)	1 (4.3%)	23 (1.2%)	39 (92.9%)	3 (7.1%)	42 (2.9%)	61 (93.8%)	4 (6.2%)	65 (2.0%)
August	212 (99.5%)	1 (0.5%)	213 (11.4%)	143 (91.1%)	14 (8.9%)	157 (10.9%)	355 (95.9%)	15 (4.1%)	370 (11.2%)
September	297 (94.3%)	18 (5.7%)	315 (16.9%)	147 (98.7%)	2 (1.3%)	149 (10.3%)	444 (95.7%)	20 (4.3%)	464 (14.0%)
October	348 (95.9%)	15 (4.1%)	363 (19.4%)	182 (94.8%)	10 (5.2%)	192 (13.3%)	530 (95.5%)	25 (4.5%)	555 (16.7%)
November	856 (94.4%)	51 (5.6%)	907 (48.5%)	809 (94.4%)	48 (5.6%)	857 (59.3%)	1665 (94.4%)	99 (5.6%)	1764 (53.2%)
Total	1780 (95.2%)	89 (4.8%)	1869 (100.0%)	1367 (94.5%)	79 (5.5%)	1446 (100.0%)	3147 (94.9%)	168 (5.1%)	3315 (100%)

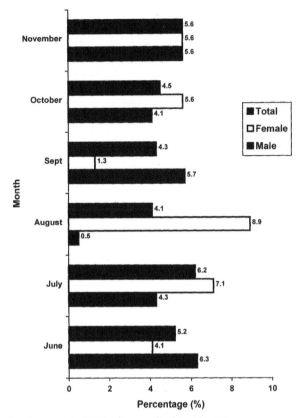

Fig. 8. Monthwise decrease in PTSD after medical treatment.

This holistic psychological intervention faced several obstacles in reaching certain populations in Kachchh. First, the existing caste system caused many problems (entry to some villages, explaining that the somatic complaints may have been caused by mental health issues, organizing camps and addressing all the people at the same platform, advising and prescribing sertraline treatment, to name a few). In addition, children were initially not counseled because of press reports erroneously suggesting that UNICEF would take care of them. Finally, accessing rescue workers was difficult, notably the military and police.

For better acceptance and results, one should integrate mental health approaches in local traditions and customs. Moreover, mental health efforts should first reach the rural areas and those without television coverage, to deliver help from disaster experts who may be the most knowledgable guides during such a crisis, and from the traditional leaders of a country such as India, from whom much more can be achieved by a few words than equivalent efforts by other authorities. Television plays a significant role in broadcasting news and current updates, informs survivors not to be scared of aftershocks as they are not true earthquakes, and plays a special role in broadcasting survival information leaflets and similar materials readied to help survivors. Finally, all of these efforts, of course, need to be rolled out in a fashion proportionate to the size of a local economy and be based on realistic and sustainable budgets. In the author's experience, funding by private agencies such as banks has

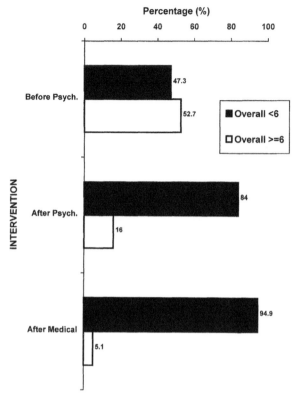

Fig. 9. Overall comparison of effect of psychological and medical intervention.

proved to be much more successful and less bureaucratic than aid agencies and governmental funding.

In the long term, the mental health program on behalf of the 2001 earthquake survivors not only raised the mental health awareness of the people in Kachchh, but has paved the way for the opening of many new mental health clinics and has increased the number of psychiatrists available to the district in a very short time. The number of psychiatrists has tripled in Kachchh since the earthquake and there are also 2 Departments of Psychiatry in Medical Colleges in this area that earlier did not exist. There are now also a few specialist counseling facilities in the 2 major cities of Kachchh.

ACKNOWLEDGMENTS

The author thanks Dr Yoep Toebosch, Dr Vijay Shah, and Dr Vidhi Patel.

REFERENCES

1. Davidson JR. Pharmacotherapy of posttraumatic stress disorder: treatment options, long-term follow-up, and predictors of outcome. J Clin Psychiatry 2000; 6(Suppl 5):52–6.
2. Baxi RK. Psycho-social aspects of earthquake affected population. 2001.

3. Ankle Ehlers. Post traumatic stress disorder, New Oxford Textbook of Psychiatry, chapter 4.6.2. Including rating scales in English.
4. Davidson JR, Connor KM. Management of posttraumatic disorder: diagnostic and therapeutic issues. J Clin Psychiatry 1999;60(Suppl 18):33–8.
5. Mahendru RK, Mahendru S. Selection of antidepressant drugs in general practice. J Indian Med Assoc 2001;99(1):54–5.

The Enduring Mental Health Impact of the September 11th Terrorist Attacks

Challenges and Lessons Learned

Fatih Ozbay, MD[a,b,c,*], Tanja Auf der Heyde, PhD[b],
Dori Reissman, MD[d], Vansh Sharma, MD[b]

KEYWORDS

- World Trade Center • Disaster response • Crisis counseling • Barriers to care
- PTSD

KEY POINTS

- Training emergency response staff to carry out potentially traumatizing tasks that normally fall outside their scope of work before a disaster or before their deployment and limiting the length of shifts and total duration of work may reduce psychiatric morbidity in disaster workers.
- Clinicians who treat disaster survivors must be familiar with the changing needs of a traumatized population over the course of time.
- Once chronic, posttraumatic stress disorder (PTSD) is a difficult condition to treat and is often comorbid with other major psychiatric disorders. Early interventions administered by well-trained, culturally and linguistically capable clinicians may prevent chronic PTSD and the myriad of comorbid psychiatric conditions that consume a substantial amount of resources in the long-term.
- In the long-term, resources should be allocated to maintain an infrastructure to continue public outreach and psychoeducation while training clinicians in advanced and evidence-based treatments to address the complex comorbidity associated with chronic PTSD.

[a] The WTC Mental Health Program, Icahn School of Medicine at Mount Sinai, New York, NY, USA; [b] Department of Psychiatry, Icahn School of Medicine at Mount Sinai, New York, NY, USA; [c] Department of Preventive Medicine, Icahn School of Medicine at Mount Sinai, New York, NY, USA; [d] The WTC Health Program, National Institute for Occupational Health and Safety, Centers for Disease Control and Prevention, Atlanta, GA, USA
* Corresponding author. The WTC Mental Health Program, Icahn School of Medicine at Mount Sinai, New York, NY.
E-mail address: fatih.ozbay@mssm.edu

Psychiatr Clin N Am 36 (2013) 417–429
http://dx.doi.org/10.1016/j.psc.2013.05.011
0193-953X/13/$ – see front matter © 2013 Elsevier Inc. All rights reserved.

psych.theclinics.com

INTRODUCTION

On September 11, 2001, terrorists affiliated with the militant group al-Qaeda hijacked and flew 2 commercial passenger planes into the north and south towers of the World Trade Center (WTC) complex in New York City,[1] resulting in the massacre of 2606 victims.[2] The September 11th attack on the WTC was the first act of war on the US mainland since the Civil War[3] and the worst man-made disaster in recent history. Tens of thousands of people were affected by the destruction of the towers and the subsequent rescue, recovery, and cleanup operations.[4]

In this article, the authors review the existing literature on the mental health impact of the September 11th attacks and the implications for disaster mental health clinicians and policy makers. The first section focuses on the demographic characteristics of those affected as well as the state of mental health needs and existing mental health delivery services. Second, the authors describe the nature of the disaster and its primary impacts on lives, infrastructure, and socioeconomic factors. The third section outlines the acute aftermath in the days and weeks after September 11, 2001 in terms of the mental health impact and initial response. Fourth, the authors portray the persistent mental health impact and evolution of services of the postacute aftermath, months to years after the attacks. The fifth and final section lists implications for future disaster mental health practitioners and policy makers.

THE PRE-EVENT COMMUNITY

In 2002, the New York City Health Department established the WTC Health Registry, a database for following people who were exposed to the dust cloud, the fumes from the fires, and the mental trauma of the terrorist attacks.[5] Murphy and colleagues[6] identified 4 exposure groups: rescue and recovery workers, residents, students and school staff, and building occupants and passersby in lower Manhattan. Of the estimated 400,000 individuals eligible for the baseline health survey, more than 71,000 interviewer-administered surveys were completed.[6] Roughly 60% of the respondents were men; 47.3% were aged between 25 and 44 years; and 63% were non-Hispanic white, 11.9% non-Hispanic black, 13.4% Hispanic, 7.5% Asian, and 4.3% other.[7] Of the respondents, 11.3% made less than $25,000 a year, 21.6% made $25,000 to $50,000, 21.1% made $50,000 to 75,000, 34% made $75,000 to 150,000, and 11.8% earned more than $150,000 a year.[7]

An estimated 40,000 to 92,000 people were involved in the rescue, recovery, and cleanup operations.[4] A subsegment of this population is served by the WTC Health Program Clinical Centers of Excellence and shows significant diversity across multiple domains (eg, profession and employment status, state of physical health, cultural identity, and immigration status). Most of the rescue and recovery workers are men, more than half of them are white, and 86% are union members.[4] A recent large-scale study[8] found that of the 27,449 participants, 86% were men, the average age of the responders was 38 years, 66% were married, 17% were single, and roughly 8% were separated or divorced. Roughly 57% identified as white, 11% as black, 31% as Hispanic, 1% as Asian, 3% as other, and 28% were unknown.[8] An earlier study[4] found that of the 10,132 participants, approximately 37% attended college, 14% had graduated college, and 7% had attended graduate school. In this sample, more than 62% had arrived within the first 48 hours of the attack; 84% began working on the sites during the first week, and 91% arrived by September 24, 2001.[4]

Several different professions were represented among the rescue and recovery workers. Protective services and military were among the largest occupational groups to respond to the attack.[8,9] Other represented professions included technical and utility workers, construction workers, asbestos cleaners, administrators, and volunteers with disaster-relief agencies, among others.[10] Wisnivesky and colleagues[8] reported that 48% of their participants (N = 27,449) worked in protective services or the military, 23% worked in construction, 7% in electrical or telecommunication repairs, 4% in transportation or material movers, 16% in other occupations, and 2% were unemployed or retired. Regarding working status at the site, 81% were workers, 11% were volunteers, and 8% both worked and volunteered. According to Katz and colleagues,[11] most of the foreign-born workers at Ground Zero were from Latin America (mainly Colombia and Ecuador) or Eastern Europe (mainly Poland).

THE ATTACK AND THE PRIMARY IMPACT

On the morning of September 11, 2001, 10 al-Qaeda agents hijacked American Airlines Flight 11 and United Airlines Flight 175 and intentionally flew the planes into the WTC towers at 8:46 AM and 9:03 AM, respectively.[12] At the time of impact, each plane was flying around 500 mph and carried approximately 10,000 gallons of jet fuel.[12] Hundreds of people were trapped above the points of impact and died of smoke inhalation and fires, whereas 200 victims jumped from the towers to escape the smoke and flames.[13] In less than 90 minutes, both towers collapsed. Thousands of tons of toxic debris from the pulverized buildings covered the WTC site, which was referred to as Ground Zero.[14] In addition to the twin towers, 2 other buildings in the WTC complex (3 WTC and 7 WTC) were completely destroyed. The remaining buildings, which included the US Customs House (6 WTC), 4 WTC, and 5 WTC, were severely damaged. The Deutsche Bank Building at 130 Liberty Street suffered structural damage and was eventually demolished.

In New York City, about 430,000 job-months, which is equivalent to 143,000 jobs, were lost as a result of the attacks.[15] Approximately 70% of the lost job-months belonged to the export sector, which also represented 86% of all lost wages ($2.8 billion dollars in the 3 months after the attacks). Investigators estimated that the gross city product in New York City declined by $27.3 billion during the last quarter of 2001 and all of 2002.[16] Zimmerman and Sherman[17] reviewed the impact of the attacks on New York City's public transportation infrastructure, and estimated that about 1800 feet of subway track were destroyed when the WTC buildings collapsed, severely limiting the availability of public transit services and crippling the Port Authority Trans Hudson Corporation's (PATH) underground rail system that connects New Jersey with Manhattan for an extended period of time.[17] However, a substantial level of Metropolitan Transit Authority service in Manhattan rebounded within hours of the attacks. In some cases, trains made use of alternative routes in the rail system, which was critical to evacuating people from Ground Zero.[17] Within 2 weeks, transit ridership was beginning to rebound, although it had not yet reached pre-September 11th levels.[18]

Survivors who were able to escape from the towers, lower Manhattan residents, and first responders had a variety of traumatic exposures. Of the 71,437 enrollees of the WTC Health Registry, 36,452 reported getting caught in the dust cloud resulting from the collapse of the towers.[7] Almost 70% of enrollees witnessed a traumatic event that day, including seeing an airplane hit the WTC towers, people jumping from the towers, buildings collapsing, people running away, and people being injured or killed.[7] A clinician first responder described his first visit to Ground Zero as an overwhelming assault on the senses, where he encountered flames, twisted steel girders, and noxious smoke billowing from the rubble.[19]

THE ACUTE AFTERMATH

The rescue and recovery workers who arrived at the site on September 11th or in the days and weeks after the attacks were also met with unprecedented physical hazards from the disintegrated structure and contents of the WTC towers, the jet fuel from the planes, and the resulting fires.[20] In addition, many of them were confronted with the loss of friends and colleagues; the process of handling dead bodies, body parts, and personal effects; and inhaling the odor of burning debris and decomposing bodies.[4] The disaster caused fear and uncertainty among the citizens of New York City; access to many residential homes, schools, and workplaces remained restricted.[21] At the national level, during the week following the attacks, 44% of the adults who were contacted by phone reported a substantial degree of stress.[22] Respondents reported that they used various strategies, such as talking with others (98%), religion (90%), participating in group activities (60%), and giving to charity (36%), to cope with stress.[22]

Immediately after the September 11th attacks, New York City was declared a federal disaster area and became eligible for programs funded by the Federal Emergency Management Agency (FEMA). One such program, the Crisis Counseling Assistance and Training Program (CCP), supports short-term interventions for those psychologically affected by large-scale disasters. New York's CCP, Project Liberty, was awarded $155 million by FEMA.[23] The New York State Office of Mental Health (NYSOMH) oversaw the governmental agencies and nongovernmental organizations (NGOs) that delivered crisis counseling and public education services to 1.2 million people between September 12, 2001, and December 30, 2004.[24] During the emergency Immediate Services Program phase, which ran from September 12, 2001 to June 12, 2002, Project Liberty provided crisis counseling services according to the CCP model, which aims to facilitate a "return to pre-disaster functioning among as many people as possible."[24] The FEMA stipulations required that recipients of services remain anonymous and did not provide funding for psychological assessment and treatment services during this critical period. In addition, the NGOs were forbidden from using some of their existing mental health professionals because of the federal antisupplantation rules,[25] which meant that the agencies had to rely on newly hired staff whose training level and qualifications may have been insufficient.

In fact, there is reason to think that in the wake of September 11th, people living in the New York area actually made *fewer* visits to mental health providers than they did during other time periods. One study probed outpatient mental health care utilization among residents of the New York metropolitan area who were enrolled in the health plans of a large insurance company.[26] During the baseline period, there was a monthly average of 75,225 outpatient mental health visits, which declined to 18% less than expected in September; this dip persisted for the next 2 quarters (14% and 13%, respectively).[26] Relative declines in mental health service use tended to be greater for residents of the innermost zone than for residents of the more distant zones. Among adult Medicaid enrollees living within a 3-mile radius of the WTC site, there was a 10% increase in the rate of behavioral and mental health diagnoses at emergency departments after September 11th compared with previous time periods.[27]

THE POSTACUTE AFTERMATH: THE PERSISTENT MENTAL HEALTH IMPACT AND EVOLUTION OF SERVICES

Schlenger and colleagues[28] administered a Web-based epidemiologic survey to a nationally representative sample 1 to 2 months after the attacks. They found that the New York City metropolitan area had the nation's highest prevalence of probable posttraumatic stress disorder (PTSD) (11.2%). To compare, Washington, DC had a rate of 2.7%, other major metropolitan areas were at 3.6%, and the rest of the country had a rate of 4.0%, although national levels of significant distress (as opposed to PTSD specifically) were within expected ranges.[28] PTSD symptom levels were associated with sex, age, and direct exposure to the attacks.

To monitor the health of those directly affected by the September 11th attacks, the WTC registry conducted 2 major surveys: the Wave 1 (2–3 years after September 11th) and Wave 2 (5–6 years after September 11th) surveys.[5] The findings show that the WTC attacks had a significant and pervasive impact on both the mental and physical health of those who were exposed. Two to 3 years after September 11th, 16% of the nearly 69,000 adults in the registry screened positive for PTSD,[5] and 8% screened positive for serious psychological distress. Among the 50,000 study participants of the Wave 2 survey, 19% reported new posttraumatic stress symptoms 5 to 6 years later, an increase from 14% in 2003 and 2004.[5] More than half (52%) of those who reported posttraumatic stress symptoms said they had not received treatment in the previous year. The rate of PTSD was highest among low-income (32%) and Hispanic enrollees (31%) and those who were passing through the area on September 11th (23%), including commuters and tourists.[5]

Several studies have traced the persistence of multiple illnesses, including mental health disorders, in WTC rescue and recovery workers and found that PTSD is associated with extensive physical and mental health comorbidities. One study measured the incidence of PTSD, depression, and panic disorders in both New York City police officers and other rescue and recovery workers.[8] In terms of preexisting mental health concerns, 1% of nonpolice rescue and recovery workers reported a history of physician-diagnosed PTSD before the WTC attacks, and 3% reported a previous diagnosis of depression.[8] The study showed that, in nonpolice rescue and recovery workers, the 9-year cumulative incidence of depression was 27.5%, PTSD was 31.9%, and panic disorder was 21.2%. PTSD had the highest cumulative incidence in both groups, and the incidence of PTSD peaked in the fourth year after September 11th for both groups.[8] Those responders with all 3 conditions (PTSD, depression, and panic disorder) outnumbered those with PTSD alone or with comorbid PTSD and depression. Studies have also shown that probable PTSD was associated with more than double the risk for an alcohol problem and more than a 17-fold risk for reported social disability.[4]

Research has revealed lower rates of full PTSD in police involved in the WTC rescue and recovery effort. Perrin and colleagues[29] reported a PTSD prevalence that ranged from 6.2% for police to 21.2% for unaffiliated volunteers. Wisnivesky and colleagues[8] also reported a lower prevalence of mental health disorders in police officers than in other rescue and recovery workers. In their study, the cumulative incidence of PTSD, panic disorder, and depression was substantially lower in the police officers group than in the other group.[8] The 9-year cumulative incidence of depression was 7.0%, PTSD was 9.3%, and panic disorder was 8.4%. The investigators stated that possible reasons for this finding include training, self-selection of highly resilient individuals in NYPD recruitment, and possible underreporting of mental health symptoms because of concerns related to repercussions.[8] As Perrin and colleagues[29] point out, police officers face graver consequences if their psychological health is in question because their job requires carrying a firearm. A study by Pietrzak and colleagues[30] highlights the importance of a more inclusive conceptualization of PTSD, particularly as it pertains to police. This study (N = 8466) found that, although full PTSD occurred at an even lower prevalence in this population than in the other reported studies (5.4%), the prevalence of subsyndromal WTC-related PTSD was 15.4%.[30]

Subsyndromal PTSD, which may result in clinically significant PTSD symptoms, was also associated with elevated rates of comorbid depression, panic disorder, alcohol abuse, somatic symptoms, and functional difficulties.[30] After the attacks, veterans with PTSD related to their military service experienced an immediate but transitory increase in their symptoms as well as longer-lasting subjective impairment.[31] Unfortunately, much about cumulative trauma remains unclear.[32]

In terms of physical health disorders, asthma, sinusitis, and gastroesophageal reflux disease had the highest cumulative incidences and also showed considerable comorbidities.[8] Holman and colleagues[33] reported that, even after adjusting for other factors, acute stress after September 11th was associated with a 53% increase in the incidence of cardiovascular ailments (over the 3 subsequent years), and people who reported high levels of acute stress right after the attacks also reported an increased incidence of hypertension and hearing problems.

Several risk factors associated with posttraumatic stress symptoms have been identified in the literature. These risk factors include pre-event psychopathology, female sex, recent immigration to the United States, and increased hours of viewing event-related media coverage.[21] Among the rescue and recovery workers, immigrants faced distinct challenges in accessing needed care, possibly because immigrants often lack an understanding of their rights to mental health care; many have a low income and lack insurance; and many, both legal and undocumented alike, may be afraid of possible immigration consequences of using services and benefits.[11]

More than a year after the attacks, and consistent with the literature reviewed earlier, findings based on the logs made by the Project Liberty providers indicated that the mental health needs of the community were beyond the scope of what could be addressed within the CCP's brief crisis counseling model.[34] In response, FEMA approved an expansion of the program to provide enhanced services to individuals who were struggling with disaster-related mental health "problems."[23] Although these anonymously provided services were informed by cognitive behavioral therapy–based interventions for anxiety and depression, it is important to note that they did not amount to comprehensive mental health assessment and treatment services for psychiatric disorders associated with trauma exposure. Because these enhanced services were not considered treatment, they did not include coverage for critical interventions, such as psychopharmacologic management, intensive outpatient treatment, substance abuse rehabilitation, and hospitalization.[24]

Barriers to mental health care were investigated by Boscarino and colleagues[35] who reported that African Americans and Hispanics were less likely than Caucasians to access treatment services. Having a primary care physician and a history of more than 2 traumatic life events predicted greater access to psychopharmacologic treatment, which was less likely to be used by ethnic minority groups.[35] Several studies indicated that a substantial number of people were suffering from PTSD, depression, and other anxiety disorders during the years following the attacks[28,36] (one reviewer estimated that there were approximately 200,000 cases of chronic PTSD at 1-year follow-up[37]). However, mental health visits declined compared with the first 2 months following September 11th.[35]

Other barriers to accessing services after the attacks included programmatic barriers (lack of program visibility and accessibility); personal barriers, such as stigmatization and unfamiliarity with September 11th–related health problems and services; lack of referrals from their primary care providers; and reluctance to connect their symptoms to the events of September 11th because of a lack of knowledge, the amount of time that had elapsed since the attacks, and the attribution of current health symptoms to the aging process.[38] Some rescue and recovery workers expressed fear of connecting their symptoms to their exposure because they thought retraumatized by the knowledge that their exposure might have caused a potentially life-threatening illness.[38]

In response to the WTC attacks, clinicians at the Mount Sinai Irving Selikoff Center for Occupational and Environmental Medicine, in partnership with other affected organizations, developed a medical screening program to evaluate the health status of rescue and recovery workers.[39] The WTC Worker and Volunteer Medical Screening Program received federal funding from the National Institute for Occupational Safety and Health (NIOSH), and examinations began in July 2002. Eligibility criteria for registering with the WTC Medical Monitoring and Treatment Program included having worked or volunteered in the capacity of rescue, recovery, restoration, or cleanup for at least 24 hours from September 11 to September 30, 2001 or for more than 80 hours from September 11 to December 31, 2001 in one or more of the following locations: Manhattan south of Canal Street, barge-loading piers in Manhattan, or the Staten Island landfill.[40] Two other groups were eligible: members of the Office of the Chief Medical Examiner who processed human remains and workers from the PATH who cleaned tunnels for 24 hours or more from September 11, 2001 to July 1, 2002. New York City firefighters were assessed and received services through a separate program.[41] The significant need for a mental health component of the program soon became apparent. In collaboration with Disaster Psychiatry Outreach, Mount Sinai School of Medicine's Department of Psychiatry obtained additional funding to implement a 1-year project to aid the medical program in evaluating the mental health status of the responders.[10] Approximately 6000 responders completed self-administered mental health questionnaires, and 3000 in-person evaluations were conducted during this period.[10] Subsequent funding by the NIOSH enabled the continuation of this assessment protocol and authorized the delivery of on-site treatment services. The WTC Mental Health Program grew out of this project. Currently, the Mental Health Program operates within the WTC Health Program at Mount Sinai School of Medicine Center of Excellence and provides ongoing psychiatric assessment and treatment services for WTC exposure-related mental health conditions.

DISCUSSION
Implications for Disaster Response Planning

Communication problems may have indirectly contributed to the loss of life and traumatic exposures immediately after the attacks, specifically by delaying the evacuation of the WTC buildings and the surrounding area.[12] Zimmerman and Sherman[17] suggest that emergency response planners should be mindful of people's tendency to seek information and other people during a disaster when they design communication and risk management policies. Future psychology research should focus on identifying additional factors that can influence emergency behavior to minimize casualties and reduce the frequency and intensity of traumatic exposures suffered by survivors and responders.

The literature suggests that workers who did not have the appropriate training for disaster-related work (such as volunteers and construction workers) had a higher risk for developing PTSD.[29] Among the personnel who had prior experience with emergency response (eg, emergency medical staff), those who performed dangerous tasks that fell outside the scope of their specific training (such as firefighting, search and rescue operations) were also at increased risk.[29] Early arrival at the WTC site, particularly on September 11, and working more than 3 months were additional risk factors.[29] Training emergency response staff to carry out potentially traumatizing tasks that normally fall outside their scope of work before a disaster or before their deployment may reduce psychiatric morbidity in this population. In order to minimize the PTSD risk, policy makers should also consider limiting the length of shifts and total duration of work for those who will participate in future disaster response efforts.

Crisis Counseling

Project Liberty was a successful public outreach, crisis-counseling, and psychoeducation program that was administered by the NYSOMH, which oversaw approximately 200 agencies that provided services to nearly 1.2 million people in New York City.[24] The project was, and remains to this day, the most expensive CCP funded by FEMA. Unfortunately, there is very little scientific evidence to suggest that the interventions supported by the CCP are effective in preventing and/or treating the various psychiatric disorders that can be caused or exacerbated by trauma exposure.[37] Furthermore, the FEMA model assumes that those who need treatment services can receive this care from public mental health systems. However, as Sederer and colleagues[24] argued, the US public mental health system had and continues to have limitations in providing patients with access to high-quality, evidence-based, and coordinated care. NYSOMH officials communicated the significant gap between the mental health needs of the affected population and the capabilities of the existing infrastructure to FEMA. In return, they were provided with additional funding to offer enhanced services, which were mainly cognitive behavioral therapy–based interventions for disaster-related stress, depression, and anxiety.[24] However, as noted earlier, these enhanced services did not amount to mental health treatment. Comprehensive psychiatric assessments by qualified, culturally and linguistically capable clinicians and basic interventions, such as sedatives for severe anxiety or antidepressants for major depression, were not available.[24] The lessons learned from these challenges should be considered to expand the CCP model to include comprehensive mental health treatment services in addition to education and crisis counseling. Several studies suggest that patients whose PTSD symptoms do not decrease within 3 to 6 months of trauma exposure become chronic cases,[42] as reflected by the current definition of PTSD in the *Diagnostic and Statistical Manual of Mental Disorders* (Fourth Edition).[43] Once chronic, PTSD is a difficult condition to treat and is often comorbid with other major psychiatric disorders.[42] On the other hand, recent literature suggests that prolonged exposure (PE) and cognitive therapy can prevent chronic PTSD in patients who develop acute stress disorder and meet the full criteria for PTSD within a few weeks of trauma exposure.[44] Crisis counseling services should be provided by adequately trained mental health clinicians and should focus on identifying and treating those who need comprehensive care.

Training Clinicians

After September 11, 2001, several community-based organizations, professional associations, hospitals, and government agencies began to provide disaster mental health training for practitioners. A review conducted by The National Center for Disaster Preparedness at Columbia University's School of Public Health indicated that the effectiveness of these programs is hard to assess.[45] A lack of a standard curriculum and a widespread lack of record keeping and credentialing of trainers were noted. To improve the quality of these training programs, Gill and Gershon[45] recommended specifying clear objectives and measureable outcomes for each program, the mandatory use of a specific training manual, and minimum criteria that all programs must meet (eg, course length, format, and instructor qualifications).

Long-term Planning

Chronic PTSD is not the only outcome associated with trauma exposure. PTSD is highly comorbid with several other disabling psychiatric disorders, such as major depression (48%), generalized anxiety disorder (17%), panic disorder (7%), alcohol abuse (52%), and substance abuse (35%).[42] The comorbidity between PTSD and major depressive disorder may be partially caused by overlapping symptoms of both disorders.[46] However, Chiu and colleagues[41] reported that, among the WTC exposed firefighters, PTSD and depression are different outcomes with specific risk factors. Conducting a meta-analysis of 20 studies, Panagioti and colleagues[47] reported that PTSD and depression equally increase the risk for suicidality.

Another condition that is commonly comorbid with PTSD, borderline personality disorder (BDP), is characterized by affect dysregulation, impulsivity, self-injurious behavior, anger, and identity disturbance.[43] Several studies indicate that this comorbidity can lead to more anxiety and depression, worse physical health,[48] greater impulsivity and suicide proneness,[49] or higher self-reported anger and anxiety symptoms.[50] An increased likelihood of suicide attempts has been found among individuals with comorbid PTSD-BPD relative to those with PTSD alone.[50] Pagura and colleagues[51] posit that multiple traumas and repetition of trauma early in life may be especially important in influencing the development of characterological vulnerabilities that may culminate in comorbid PTSD-BPD. They also maintain that PTSD and BPD have a high degree of lifetime co-occurrence but are not entirely overlapping. Because this concurrence is associated with poorer functioning compared with either diagnosis alone, the researchers emphasize the clinical utility of diagnosing both conditions.[51] Evidence-based treatments, such as dialectical behavioral therapy (DBT), mentalization-based treatment, and transference-focused psychotherapy, should be made available to address the needs of this complex and clinically challenging subpopulation of patients with PTSD. A recent study demonstrated that PE can be integrated with DBT to treat PTSD in suicidal and self-injuring individuals with BPD without causing exacerbations of self-injurious behavior or crisis service use.[52]

There is extensive literature indicating that alcohol and substance abuse/dependence disorders are also common among patients with PTSD.[53] The treatment of these conditions requires infrastructure to provide patients with rapid access to outpatient or inpatient detoxification, residential rehabilitation, and intensive outpatient treatment services that should delivered by highly trained multidisciplinary teams consisting of addiction psychiatrists, nurses, case workers, substance abuse counselors, and family therapists.

In summary, clinicians who treat disaster survivors must be familiar with the changing needs of a traumatized population over the course of the days, weeks, months, and years following the event. During the acute period, resources should be focused on identifying and reaching out to individuals who are symptomatic. Policy makers should consider integrating this triaging system with specialized treatment services, which should also be covered as part of the disaster relief efforts. Early interventions administered by well-trained, culturally and linguistically capable clinicians may prevent chronic PTSD and the myriad of comorbid psychiatric conditions that consume a substantial amount of resources in the long-term. The complex comorbidity associated with chronic PTSD requires highly specialized treatments that are scarcely available. In the long-term, resources should be allocated to maintain an infrastructure to continue public outreach and psychoeducation while training clinicians in these advanced and evidence-based treatments. Quality-assurance (QA) procedures should be implemented to ensure that only competent and adequately trained mental health clinicians provide these professional services. QA measures should be defined for every stage of disaster response and should be captured in a way that can be quickly used to improve performance as well as facilitate scientific research. As discussed earlier, NGOs that are funded via FEMA's CCP-based projects are not allowed to use their existing staff in disaster relief efforts because of the federal antisupplantation rules. Although these rules ensure that CCPs do not disrupt the provision of routine services, they also prevent the utilization of the most experienced and well-trained staff, leaving the extremely challenging disaster mental health work to individuals who may not be sufficiently qualified to render them. Policy makers should consider revising these rules to introduce a level of flexibility to ensure that highly trained clinicians can be used to address disaster-related mental health issues. In conclusion, the treatment of chronic PTSD and comorbid disorders presents particular challenges that necessitate new and creative collaborative approaches for best outcomes, both for the continued treatment of patients currently suffering from these disorders and to ensure better service provisions in the future.

REFERENCES

1. Cruz MA, Burger R, Keim M. The first 24 hours of the World Trade Center attacks of 2001–the Centers for Disease Control and Prevention emergency phase response. Prehospital Disaster Med 2007;22(6):473–7.
2. Terry Frieden CK. Accused 9/11 plotter Khalid Sheikh Mohammed faces New York trial. CNN 2009;2013(13):1.
3. Acosta JK, Levenson RL Jr. Observations from ground zero at the World Trade Center in New York City, part II: theoretical and clinical considerations. Int J Emerg Ment Health 2002;4(2):119–26.
4. Stellman JM, Smith RP, Katz CL, et al. Enduring mental health morbidity and social function impairment in World Trade Center rescue, recovery, and cleanup workers: the psychological dimension of an environmental health disaster. Environ Health Perspect 2008;116(9):1248–53.
5. Brackbill RM, Hadler JL, DiGrande L, et al. Asthma and posttraumatic stress symptoms 5 to 6 years following exposure to the World Trade Center terrorist attack. J Am Med Assoc 2009;302(5):502–16.
6. Murphy J, Brackbill RM, Thalji L, et al. Measuring and maximizing coverage in the World Trade Center Health Registry. Stat Med 2007;26(8):1688–701.
7. Farfel M, DiGrande L, Brackbill R, et al. An overview of 9/11 experiences and respiratory and mental health conditions among World Trade Center Health Registry enrollees. J Urban Health 2008;85(6):880–909.
8. Wisnivesky JP, Teitelbaum SL, Todd AC, et al. Persistence of multiple illnesses in World Trade Center rescue and recovery workers: a cohort study. Lancet 2011; 378(9794):888–97.
9. Pietrzak RH, Goldstein MB, Malley JC, et al. Structure of posttraumatic stress disorder symptoms and psychosocial functioning in Veterans of Operations Enduring Freedom and Iraqi Freedom. Psychiatry Res 2010;178(2):323–9.
10. Katz CL, Smith R, Silverton M, et al. A mental health program for ground zero rescue and recovery workers: cases and observations. Psychiatr Serv 2006; 57(9):1335–8.
11. Katz CL, Jutras-Aswad D, Kiliman M, et al. Alcohol Use in polish 9/11 responders: implications for cross-cultural treatment. J Psychiatr Pract 2012; 18(1):55–63.

12. Kean T, Hamilton L, Ben-Veniste R, et al. The 9/11 commission report: final report of the national commission on terrorist attacks upon the United States (9/11 Report) 2004;Y 3.2:T 27/2/FINAL.
13. Cauchon D, Moore M. Desperation forced a horrific decision. USA Today 2002.
14. Gates A. Buildings rise from rubble while health crumbles. The New York Times 2006.
15. Dolfman ML, Wasser SF. 9/11 and the New York City economy: a borough-by-borough analysis. Mon Labor Rev 2004;127(6):3–33.
16. Makinen G. The economic effects of 9/11: a retrospective assessment. 2002;RL31617.
17. Zimmerman R, Sherman MF. To leave an area after disaster: how evacuees from the WTC buildings left the WTC area following the attacks. Risk Anal 2011;31(5): 787–804.
18. Zimmerman R, Simonoff JS. Transportation density and opportunities for expediting recovery to promote security. J Appl Secur Res 2009;4(1–2):48–59.
19. Levenson RL Jr, Acosta JK. Observations from ground zero at the World Trade Center in New York City, part I. Int J Emerg Ment Health 2001;3(4):241–4.
20. Landrigan PJ, Lioy PJ, Thurston G, et al. Health and environmental consequences of the World Trade Center disaster. Environ Health Perspect 2004; 112(6):731–9.
21. Perlman SE, Friedman S, Galea S, et al. Short-term and medium-term health effects of 9/11. Lancet 2011;378(9794):925–34.
22. Schuster MA, Stein BD, Jaycox LH, et al. A national survey of stress reactions after the September 11, 2001, terrorist attacks. N Engl J Med 2001;345(20): 1507–12.
23. Donahue SA, Jackson CT, Shear KM, et al. Outcomes of enhanced counseling services provided to adults through project liberty. Psychiatr Serv 2006;57(9): 1298–303.
24. Sederer LI, Lanzara CB, Essock SM, et al. Lessons learned from the New York State mental health response to the September 11, 2001, attacks. Psychiatr Serv 2011;62(9):1085–9.
25. Gomes C, McGuire TG, Foster MJ, et al. Did project liberty displace community-based Medicaid services in New York? Psychiatr Serv 2006;57(9):1309–12.
26. Green DC, Buehler JW, Silk BJ, et al. Trends in healthcare use in the New York City region following the terrorist attacks of 2001. Biosecur Bioterror 2006;4(3): 263–75.
27. DiMaggio C, Galea S, Richardson LD. Emergency department visits for behavioral and mental health care after a terrorist attack. Ann Emerg Med 2007;50(3): 327–34.
28. Schlenger WE, Caddell JM, Ebert L. Psychological reactions to terrorist attacks: findings from the national study of Americans' reactions to September 11. JAMA 2002;4(3):119.
29. Perrin MA, DiGrande L, Wheeler K, et al. Differences in PTSD prevalence and associated risk factors among World Trade Center disaster rescue and recovery workers. Am J Psychiatry 2007;164(9):1385–94.
30. Pietrzak RH, Schechter CB, Bromet EJ, et al. The burden of full and subsyndromal posttraumatic stress disorder among police involved in the World Trade Center rescue and recovery effort. J Psychiatr Res 2012;46(7):835–42.
31. Niles BL, Wolf EJ, Kutter CJ. Posttraumatic stress disorder symptomatology in Vietnam Veterans before and after September 11. J Nerv Ment Dis 2003; 191(10):682–4.

32. Franz VA, Glass CR, Arnkoff DB, et al. The impact of the September 11th terrorist attacks on psychiatric patients: a review. Clin Psychol Rev 2009; 29(4):339–47.

33. Holman EA, Silver RC, Poulin M, et al. Terrorism, acute stress, and cardiovascular health: a 3-year national study following the September 11th attacks. Arch Gen Psychiatry 2008;65(1):73–80.

34. Donahue SA, Lanzara CB, Felton CJ, et al. Project Liberty: New York's crisis counseling program created in the aftermath of September 11, 2001. Psychiatr Serv 2006;57(9):1253–8.

35. Boscarino JA, Galea S, Adams RE, et al. Mental health service and medication use in New York City after the September 11, 2001, terrorist attack. Psychiatr Serv 2004;55(3):274–83.

36. Silver RC, Holman EA, McIntosh DN, et al. Nationwide longitudinal study of psychological responses to September 11. J Am Med Assoc 2002;288(10): 1235–44.

37. Henley R, Marshall R, Vetter S. Integrating mental health services into humanitarian relief responses to social emergencies, disasters, and conflicts: a case study. J Behav Health Serv Res 2011;38(1):132–41.

38. Welch AE, Caramanica K, Debchoudhury I, et al. A qualitative examination of health and health care utilization after the September 11th terror attacks among world trade center health registry enrollees. BMC Public Health 2012;12(1):721.

39. Moline JM, Herbert R, Levin S, et al. WTC medical monitoring and treatment program: comprehensive health care response in aftermath of disaster. Mt Sinai J Med 2008;75(2):67–75.

40. Herbert R, Moline J, Skloot G, et al. The World Trade Center disaster and the health of workers: five-year assessment of a unique medical screening program. Environ Health Perspect 2006;114(12):1853–8.

41. Chiu S, Niles JK, Webber MP, et al. Evaluating risk factors and possible mediation effects in posttraumatic depression and posttraumatic stress disorder comorbidity. Public Health Rep 2011;126(2):201–9.

42. Kessler RC, Sonnega A, Bromet E, et al. Posttraumatic stress disorder in the National Comorbidity Survey. Arch Gen Psychiatry 1995;52(12):1048–60.

43. American Psychiatric Association. Task force on DSM-IV. Diagnostic and statistical manual of mental disorders: DSM-IV: international version with ICD-10 codes. Washington, DC: American Psychiatric Association; 1995.

44. Shalev AY, Ankri Y, Israeli-Shalev Y, et al. Prevention of posttraumatic stress disorder by early treatment: results from the Jerusalem Trauma Outreach And Prevention study. Arch Gen Psychiatry 2012;69(2):166–76.

45. Gill KB, Gershon RR. Disaster mental health training programmes in New York City following September 11, 2001. Disasters 2010;34(3):608–18.

46. Blanchard EB, Buckley TC, Hickling EJ, et al. Posttraumatic stress disorder and comorbid major depression: is the correlation an illusion? J Anxiety Disord 1998; 12(1):21–37.

47. Panagioti M, Gooding PA, Tarrier N. A meta-analysis of the association between posttraumatic stress disorder and suicidality: the role of comorbid depression. Compr Psychiatry 2012;53(7):915–30.

48. Bolton EE, Mueser KT, Rosenberg SD. Symptom correlates of posttraumatic stress disorder in clients with borderline personality disorder. Compr Psychiatry 2006;47(5):357–61.

49. Zlotnick C, Johnson DM, Yen S, et al. Clinical features and impairment in women with borderline personality disorder (BPD) with posttraumatic stress disorder

(PTSD), BPD without PTSD, and other personality disorders with PTSD. J Nerv Ment Dis 2003;191(11):706–13.

50. Heffernan K, Cloitre M. A comparison of posttraumatic stress disorder with and without borderline personality disorder among women with a history of childhood sexual abuse: etiological and clinical characteristics. J Nerv Ment Dis 2000;188(9):589–95.

51. Pagura J, Stein MB, Bolton JM, et al. Comorbidity of borderline personality disorder and posttraumatic stress disorder in the U.S. population. J Psychiatr Res 2010;44(16):1190–8.

52. Harned MS, Korslund KE, Foa EB, et al. Treating PTSD in suicidal and self-injuring women with borderline personality disorder: development and preliminary evaluation of a dialectical behavior therapy prolonged exposure protocol. Behav Res Ther 2012;50(6):381–6.

53. Vlahov D, Galea S, Resnick H, et al. Increased use of cigarettes, alcohol, and marijuana among Manhattan, New York, residents after the September 11th terrorist attacks. Am J Epidemiol 2002;155(11):988–96.

The 2010 Haiti Earthquake Response

Giuseppe Raviola, MD, MPH[a,b,c],*, Jennifer Severe, MD[b,d],
Tatiana Therosme, BA[d], Cate Oswald, MPH[b],
Gary Belkin, MD, PhD, MPH[e,f], Father Eddy Eustache, MA[d]

KEYWORDS

- Haiti • Earthquake • Disaster • Mental health • Psychosocial

KEY POINTS

- Mental health and disorder have generally been addressed in Haiti through traditional healing practices and religion.
- The devastating 2010 Haiti earthquake highlighted a lack of preexisting formal biomedical mental health services.
- Fragmentation and poor collaboration and communication among multiple nongovernmental entities, in the context of a disempowered central government, have defined humanitarian action in Haiti, including in the health sector.
- The earthquake has been a catalyst for the identification and integration of mental health as an integral part of the post-earthquake Haitian health care system, lack of resources notwithstanding.
- Innovative care delivery models are needed to build a mental health system of care. The development of long-term services should integrate strong traditional perceptions and beliefs, religious influences, and contemporary biopsychosocial approaches.

Disclosure: Dr Belkin is funded in part by the Sanofi Aventis Access to Medicines Program.
[a] Program in Global Mental Health and Social Change, Department of Global Health and Social Medicine, Harvard Medical School, 641 Huntington Avenue, Boston, MA 02115, USA; [b] Partners In Health, 888 Commonwealth Avenue, Boston, MA 02215, USA; [c] Psychiatry Quality Program, Boston Children's Hospital, 300 Longwood Avenue, Boston, MA 02115, USA; [d] Zanmi Lasante, Route National #3, Cange, Haiti; [e] Program in Global Mental Health, Department of Psychiatry, New York University School of Medicine, 550 First Avenue, New York, NY 10016, USA; [f] Office of Behavioral Health, New York City Health and Hospitals Corporation, 125 Worth Street, Room 423, New York, NY 10013, USA
* Corresponding author. Department of Global Health and Social Medicine, Harvard Medical School, 641 Huntington Avenue, Boston, MA 02115.
E-mail address: giuseppe_raviola@hms.harvard.edu

Psychiatr Clin N Am 36 (2013) 431–450
http://dx.doi.org/10.1016/j.psc.2013.05.006
0193-953X/13/$ – see front matter © 2013 Elsevier Inc. All rights reserved.

INTRODUCTION
Background on the Pre-Event Society

On January 12, 2010, a major earthquake struck the country of Haiti, destroying its capital, Port-au-Prince as well as a significant part of southern Haiti, and causing massive casualties. Haiti is located in the American continent, in the Caribbean Ocean, occupying one-third of the island known as Hispaniola, the Dominican Republic occupying the other two-thirds. After the United States, Haiti is the second oldest independent country in the Western Hemisphere and the first black republic, where slaves revolted against their colonial masters and declared independence in 1804. While its revolutionary past serves as a source of pride, hope, and inspiration, the oppressive legacy of slavery and subsequent exploitation has continued to mark the course of a nation whose Enlightenment ideals were compromised by residual proslavery sentiment and racism. To date, the destiny of Haiti has to a significant degree been dictated by foreign powers, whether under slavery and colonialism until revolutionary independence from France in 1804 or thereafter, as a dependent peripheral state subject to the struggle of those foreign powers for ascendancy in the Haitian economy.[1] Since the nineteenth century socioeconomic disparities have fomented divisions between elites and peasants, as long-lasting sequelae of the colonial system.[1] In this context humanitarian organizations have found a fertile ground for growth and development.

Called the "Pearl of the Antilles" in the late fifteenth century, in the years before the earthquake Haiti became the poorest nation in the Western hemisphere, with a population of 9.8 million people. Plagued by decades of political instability, social crisis, and isolation, historically Haiti has been vulnerable to natural hazards (tropical cyclones, flooding, and mudslides) but its poverty has amplified the vulnerability of its people to these events. In 2008 alone Haiti experienced 4 major storms, 1 of which killed approximately 3000 people in Gonaives. These storms together wiped out 70% of Haiti's crops, resulting in the death of many children from malnutrition in the following months.[2]

Culture, Religion, and Mental Health

In 2010 the World Health Organization (WHO) and Pan-American Health Organization (PAHO) published a literature review of culture and mental health in Haiti, a useful initial reference for those unfamiliar with mental health in the Haitian context.[3] Although French is an official language, the principal spoken language is Creole, used by about 90% of the people. About 50% of the population is illiterate. Religion plays a crucial role in all spheres of life in Haiti, including politics, morality, and health.[3–5] Religious practices in Haiti help people to cope with psychological and emotional problems, and provide an informal system of healing parallel to the biomedical health care system.[3] Religion in Haiti offers a sense of purpose, consolation, belonging, structure, and discipline, thus increasing self-esteem, alleviating despair, and providing hope.[3,6] Religious and spiritual leaders have historically been trusted by the population more readily than conventional medical institutions or mental health professionals. With increasing access to more formal mental health services since the earthquake, people have started to understand the potential usefulness of such services.

Haiti is characterized by religious diversity, including Catholicism, voodoo (which combines West African traditions and Catholicism), and various Protestant traditions. Faiths have evolved in Haiti, interacting with each other and sharing key symbolic elements.[3,7] The term "voodoo," which Americans have come to think of as something dangerous or secret, refers to an important and open part of Haitian religious life.[8]

Voodoo in Haiti is widespread and is practiced by the majority, including among Haitians who consider themselves Catholics, and to a lesser extent among Protestants.[3,9] The name voodoo comes from the word meaning *spirit*. The Black Code enacted by Louis XIV in 1685 mandated the conversion of slaves to Catholicism. In an effort to hide their religious practices, which were prohibited, slaves identified their African deities with the saints of the Catholic Church. The slaves were then able to practice a strict adhesion to Catholicism while retaining aspects of their West African religion, manifesting as voodoo.[3,5] With regard to health, it has been noted that the Western understanding of health, illness, and care is "anthropocentric," with the person considered as the center of the universe, as opposed to a "cosmocentric" vision in Haiti, of the person belonging to a vast universe of spirits, ancestors, and the natural world, all of which must be in harmony for good health.[3,10] This framework provides important background for consideration of the role of Western mental health concepts in the Haitian context, given that traditional belief systems can be considered an important informal (nonbiomedical) system of health care.

Socioeconomic Status

Haiti has suffered from a complex situation characterized by a history of foreign exploitation, high levels of rural and urban poverty with marked income inequality, strong internal divisions by class, weak governance structures, organized crime, sporadic outbreaks of violence, and alarming levels of environmental degradation.[11,12] Nearly half the population lives in extreme poverty, with unemployment reaching more than 50% in metropolitan areas. Before the earthquake, Haiti was the poorest nation in the Western hemisphere, ranked 145th of 169 countries on the Human Development Index.[13] Almost 70% of Haiti's people are younger than 30 years.[13] In 2003, nearly 60% of the population lived in rural areas.[3] The nation's capital, Port-au-Prince, is the largest city (estimated population 2,000,000 people) and the economic center of the country, with a large percentage of these people living in shacks and in extreme urban poverty.[8] Other cities are Cap Haitian (600,000 people) on the northern coast and Gonaives (34,000 people) on the northwest coast. Life expectancy is short and infant mortality is high, about 12% of children dying before their first birthday and one-third of all children dying before their fifth birthday.[8] Most houses have no running water (33% only in Port-au-Prince) with significant differentiations according to place of residence, type of housing, and level of income. Residents of rural areas generally have little access to facilities and basic services. The majority of households in Haiti do not have access to electricity, particularly in rural areas.[14,15] "Brain drain" has also affected the country's situation of vulnerability. Approximately 80% of Haiti's university graduates have left the country, with concerns also of a brain drain from the government to nongovernmental sector within the country.[16,17]

Haiti is particularly susceptible to flooding because of large-scale deforestation on the Haitian half of the island, where most trees have been cut down to make charcoal for cooking.[8] Without trees to slow or stop rainfall, the water runs over the sun-baked ground, filling low spots.[8] The climate of Haiti depends on season, terrain, and location, with rainfall occurring between April and November, and hurricanes with torrential rain and destructive wind a threat in the late summer and fall.[8] In the recent past Haiti had been able to produce enough food to adequately feed its population, but trade liberalization, food aid, and the rice-dumping phenomenon—the importation of cheaper rice from the US rather than use of locally produced rice—have slowed farming activities, pushing peasants to leave rural areas for cities where unemployment rates have been high.[18] This migration has primed the country for imminent threat of social unrest, and has also affected the food habits of Haitians, now more used to imported food than locally produced food.

Formal Mental Health Services

In 2011 WHO/PAHO published an overview of mental health services in Haiti, a useful initial reference on the subject.[14] The formal (biomedical) health care system in Haiti can be divided into 4 sectors[3]:

1. Public institutions administered by the government Ministry of Public Health and Population (MSPP); mostly unequipped and underprovided. About 1% of the total health budget is allocated for mental health[14]
2. The private nonprofit sector, comprising nongovernmental organizations (NGOs) and religious organizations
3. The mixed nonprofit sector, where staff is paid by the government but management is performed by the private sector, and unlikely to expand given the small budget of MSPP
4. The private for-profit sector, which includes physicians, dentists, nurses, and other specialists working predominantly in private practice or in clinics in urban centers

The MSPP is responsible for the health of the population, delivery of services, policy making, and management of the health budget, which makes up 7% of total public spending.[19] The public sector comprises about 36% of health facilities, and most institutions are autonomous, with no networks of services. The private sector is estimated to provide one-third of the medical care in Haiti. In 2001 there were estimated to be 2500 physicians in Haiti, of whom 88% were practicing in the country's West department including Port-au-Prince.[3,19] Most people value biomedical health care services, but are unable to access care because of structural barriers such as cost, distance, and location.[3] Given the lack of official resources allocated to health care, Haitians have learned to deal with mental health problems using different strategies common to resource-poor regions, involving traditional practitioners or religious healers as the closest and most affordable providers to cope with mental health problems. While biomedical mental health services have remained relatively undeveloped in Haiti, community-based systems of mental health care have existed for hundreds of years.

Haitian culture provides a range of explanations for illness drawing on commonly held cultural, religious, and social beliefs.[3] A variety of explanatory models can determine help-seeking behavior and use of services. Traditional practitioner structures provide care to a significant proportion of the population. There are several types of traditional healers in Haiti who treat specific diseases or attend to general well-being[3]: dokte fey or medsen fey ("leaf doctors" or herbalists), often treating illnesses such as colds, worms, diarrhea, and stomach ache; houngan or manbo (voodoo priests or priestesses), treating many conditions; dokte zo ("bone setters"), treating musculoskeletal conditions; pikirist ("injectionists"), administering parenteral preparations of herbal or Western medicine; and Fanm Saj (midwives), providing perinatal and natal care.[20] Interaction between biomedical primary care and traditional or alternative care providers are not formalized; however, some cooperation between doctors and traditional practitioners exists and in some cases has been promoted, given that they sometimes treat the same patients.[3] When faced with mental health problems, most Haitians make use of traditional practitioners or religious healers. The houngan's major role is medical, using both an extensive knowledge of herbalism and the use of diagnostic rituals as central to healing in voodoo.[3,21] Houngans search for "nonphysical" or "supernatural" causation of sickness, explained as a punishment for failing to serve the spirits, or *loa* properly, or a curse.[3,21] In general, houngans are not opposed to biomedical treatments and may refer patients whose cases are beyond their scope of expertise. It can be perceived among the population that referral decisions occur only after the client has spent money on traditional care, with the houngan perceived as exploiting the patient. The lack of alternatives, however, maintains the status quo.

Individuals use resources pragmatically, and often hold multiple or hybrid models of health and illness. As a result, the same person may seek help from multiple sources when available.[3] Haitians divide illnesses generally into several broad categories, including: maladi Bondye (God's disease, of "natural" origin); maladi moun voye sou moun (magic spells sent because of human greed, sent to punish others, or sent for revenge; a curse, spell, or hex); and those of supernatural origin, maladi lwa ("disease from the spirits").[22] Many Haitians also use a humoral theory of health and illness, with imbalance of hot and cold within the body believed to be the cause of natural illness.[3] These imbalances can stem from environmental elements such as rain, wind, sun, and dew, or emotional reactions to the physical environment (eg, witnessing lightning strike) or the actions of others.[3] Health may be restored through the use of herbal teas, regulated diet, compresses, baths, and massages. The treatment must be in the opposite direction of the imbalance to restore equilibrium. Moderate and chronic illnesses are often treated within the family or the naturally occurring social support system. Severe illnesses such as human immunodeficiency virus (HIV) and tuberculosis were originally perceived also as a result of a curse, until people learned that biomedical treatments were effective. Since that time, perceptions have very gradually shifted such that these conditions are considered to be most effectively treated by physicians and nurses.[3]

People often rely on their inner spiritual and religious strength to deal with their problems. For some people, mental health problems, problems in daily functioning, and academic underachievement are attributed to supernatural forces.[3] In such cases people generally do not blame themselves for their illness or see themselves as defective. Indeed, the sense of self may even be enhanced as a curse is often aimed at a person deemed to be attractive, intelligent, and successful.[3] This mechanism can avoid the burden of stigma in the community, whether from infectious disease or mental disorder. Mentally ill people may be seen as victims of powerful forces beyond their control, and thus receive the support of the community. Shame may be associated with the decline in functioning in severe mental illness, and the family may be reluctant to acknowledge that a member is ill.[3,23] Mental illness is also sometimes attributed to failure to please spirits, including those of deceased family members. This external attribution may help recovery, in that people can call on the spirits to intervene on their behalf to assist healing.[24] For example, the lack of proper burial and the use of mass graves following the earthquake was a phenomenon unusual in the Haitian context, but also problematic from the perspective of the experience of healthy grieving and the promotion of resilience.

At first glance it would appear that the field of psychiatry and biomedical mental health services has remained relatively undeveloped in Haiti. It has been a primarily urban phenomenon, particularly in Port-au-Prince. As in other low-income countries, before the earthquake "mental health" as defined by Western psychiatry and psychology had not been a major priority for the government in comparison with other pressing health issues such as HIV, tuberculosis, or maternal and child health. However, oversimplified conceptualizations of Haitian mental health services before the earthquake as either mostly voodoo-centric or undeveloped belie a rich and complex cultural intellectual tradition of Haitian psychiatry.[3,25,26] Formal biomedical mental health services developed historically on the initiative of Louis Price Mars and an American psychiatrist, Nathan S. Kline, who in 1959 opened the Centre Hospitalier Universitaire de Psychiatrie (University Hospital Center of Psychiatry) Mars and Kline (CHUP/MK) with the financial assistance of 3 US pharmaceutical companies, Haitian philanthropists, and the commitment of the government of President Francois Duvalier.[3] The center was first headed by Dr Mars. A tentative plan for organization of mental health services was initiated by the neuropsychiatrist Legrand Bijoux in 1975.[14] Although there was a time of promise for Haitian psychiatry, with the deterioration of the health system the quality of mental health care also gradually deteriorated. Despite the many initiatives of Drs Mars, Bijoux, and others from the 1940s to the 1960s to develop a mental health sector within MSPP, the country still does not have a national mental health plan or policy, or a system for monitoring and evaluation or epidemiologic research in mental health.[14] Haiti has had no national policy or strategy for mental health despite the different sources of trauma experienced by the country over the last 10 years that relate to socioeconomic and political violence, social insecurity, recent climate phenomena, and the cholera epidemic.[14] Following the earthquake, the MSPP interim plan for the health sector (April 2010–September 2011) did call for attention to people suffering from psychological problems.[27] The human rights of those suffering from mental illness and of the psychiatrically hospitalized have not been adequately protected by law.[14] Reliable data on the prevalence of mental disorders in Haiti are still not available.[14]

Human resources in mental health were scarce prior to the earthquake, although there remains a lack of clarity on the exact number of providers. A 2003 WHO/PAHO report counted 10 psychiatrists and 9 psychiatric nurses working in the public sector, although recent reports have suggested higher numbers.[3,14] Moreover, these professionals mostly work in Port-au-Prince, to which people must travel to receive formal mental health services. The formal mental health system has suffered from this overcentralized and underresourced system. There are 2 psychiatric hospitals in and near Port-au-Prince, CHUP/MK and Beudet, both of which were in a dilapidated state both before and after the earthquake. Between them there are approximately 180 (60 + 120) hospital beds in total.[14] Both were damaged extensively during the earthquake, reducing their operational capacity. The distribution of diagnoses observed in the psychiatric hospitals has been estimated at: schizophrenia (50%), bipolar disorder with mania (30%), other psychoses (15%), and epilepsy (5%).[14] These figures are no different from those of hospitalized patient populations in other countries, and give no idea of the real prevalence of these disorders in the community.[14] Generalist physicians are able to prescribe psychotropic drugs; however, no national formulary or treatment protocols for mental disorders exist. Formal training is also limited. As a result, generalist physicians have been reluctant to prescribe medication and prefer to refer patients to the 2 psychiatric centers for care. The availability of follow-up care in the community is very limited. In the nation's second-largest city of Cap Haitian, it has been reported that psychiatric services are limited to a monthly visit by a psychiatrist from Port-au-Prince.[3]

THE EARTHQUAKE
Event Details

On January 12, 2010 a 7.0-magnitude earthquake struck near Port-au-Prince, with strong effects felt within a 40-mile radius and the entire nation physically shaken (**Fig. 1**). At least 220,000 people were killed, with more than 300,000 injured and 1.5 million displaced and homeless.[28,29] More than 105,000 homes were destroyed and 188,000 houses were badly damaged.[29] In Port-au-Prince, 25% of civil servants died, and 60% of government and administrative buildings and 80% of schools were destroyed, including 28 of 29 government ministries (**Fig. 2**).[30] Sixty percent of schools in the South and West Departments were also destroyed or damaged.[30] Many of the 1.5 million displaced moved to establish makeshift tents, with more than 100,000 at critical risk of storms and flooding.[30] Around Port-au-Prince internally displaced person (IDP) settlements began to develop within days of the disaster (**Figs. 3** and **4**). Although not directly related to the earthquake, the cholera outbreak of October 2010 caused additional challenges to aid. In 2011 the source of the cholera outbreak was traced to a United Nations (UN) battalion from Nepal (**Fig. 5**).[31] Nine months after the outbreak, approximately 6000 people had died and more than 200,000 were infected.[30] This marks the worst cholera outbreak in recent history, as well as the best-documented cholera outbreak in modern public health.[30,32] By 2012, 7700 people had been killed and 620,000 infected, with only 17% of Haitians having access to improved sanitation and clean water, conditions that fuel the spread of the disease.[33]

Post-Earthquake Response

Mental health needs

In the acute aftermath of the earthquake there was little capacity, within either the government services or humanitarian sectors, to evaluate immediate mental health impact and response. In the weeks and months following the earthquake several groups began to be identified as being particularly vulnerable to mental health problems.[34–39] These people included survivors, those who sustained physical injuries and amputations, IDPs, children in need of protection, and those at risk of gender-based violence.[40–44] The earthquake's effects extended to those who had preexisting mental disorder, those with significant prior histories of loss and trauma, those living in the Haitian diaspora, and health care providers and others who responded to the earthquake relief effort and continued to provide ongoing services in IDP settlements, hospitals, clinics, and communities (**Fig. 6**).[45–50] The 2 psychiatric hospitals suffered significant damage. Perimeter walls at CHUP/MK collapsed, with some patients leaving the hospital and wandering the neighborhood; however, the hospital's psychiatrists set up emergency outpatient services for those presenting to the hospital, and worked courageously to support those in needs of services and living temporarily on the hospital grounds (**Fig. 7**). By the end of 2010 approximately 1.3 million people were displaced, including 380,000 children, spread across more than 1300 settlement sites.[42,51,52] Many had been seriously injured in the earthquake and required ongoing medical services.

Mental health response

Immediate psychosocial assistance activities and mental health services were largely performed by NGOs and the small number of mental health professionals in the country.[14] In the weeks following the earthquake, efforts were made to organize mental health and psychosocial responses of NGOs working in Haiti in collaboration with the Haitian government and under MSPP through the UN Cluster approach, and in accordance with the Sphere Standards and the recommendations of the Inter-Agency Standing Committee (IASC) (**Box 1**).[53]

In 2007 the IASC developed a set of guidelines for mental health and psychosocial response in complex emergencies based on a "do no harm" approach, which served as a point of reference for organizations responding to the earthquake in Haiti.[54,55] Initial response efforts included organization of religious mourning ceremonies, the application of "psychological first aid", and mobilization of resources and personnel

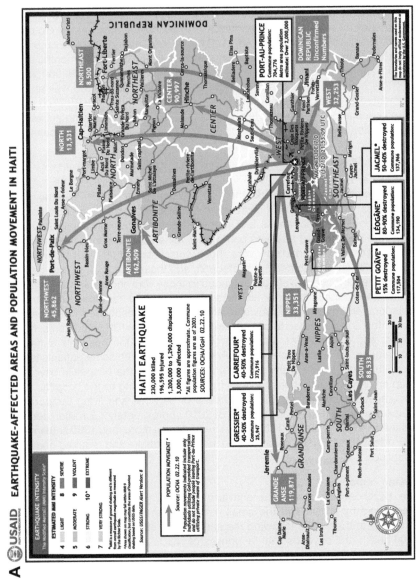

Fig. 1. United States Agency for International Development map. (A) Earthquake-affected areas and population movement in Haiti. (B) US Government humanitarian assistance to Haiti for the earthquake. A larger version of these maps is available at www.psych.theclinics.com. *Courtesy of* US Agency for International Development (http://www.usaid.gov/).

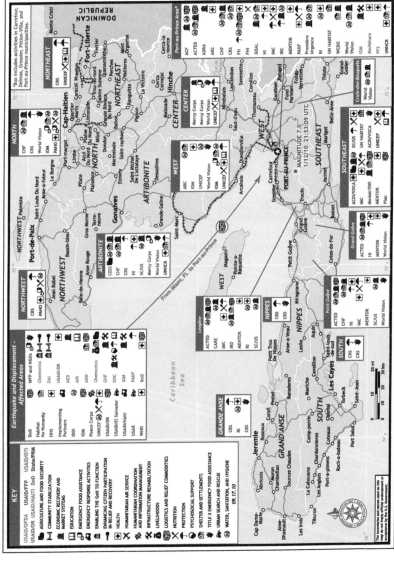

Fig. 1. (continued)

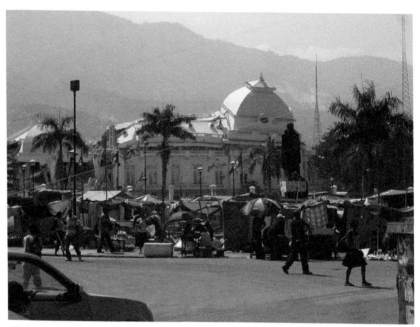

Fig. 2. Presidential palace, Port-Au-Prince (February 2010, G. Raviola). Haiti's National Palace, completed in 1920, was severely damaged in the earthquake, and razed in 2012.

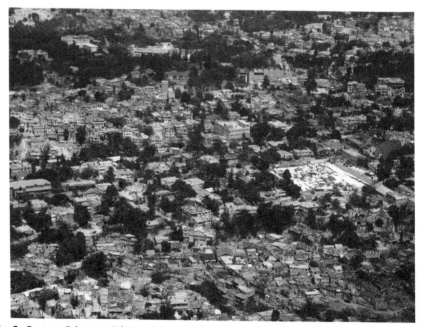

Fig. 3. Port-au-Prince aerial view (March 2010, G. Raviola). A view of Port-au-Prince from Petionville, Haiti. Soon after the earthquake, open spaces in Port-au-Prince became occupied by tented camps known as internally displaced person (IDP) settlements.

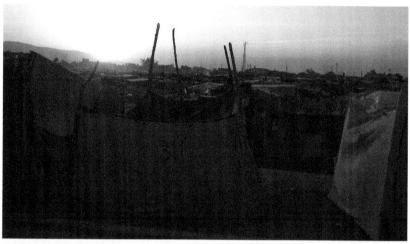

Fig. 4. IDP settlement (February 2010, G. Raviola). The Parc Jean Marie Vincent IDP settlement, Port-au-Prince, Haiti. Those living in IDP settlements have been vulnerable to illness, violence, rains, and flooding.

to support those in extreme distress (**Figs. 8** and **9**).[12] Responding organizations provided a range of services in the immediate emergency and the months following.

Within MSPP a Haitian national mental health authority was appointed to coordinate government activities on policy, mental health legislation, and the planning of services, as well as to direct the cluster. WHO and PAHO engaged in a role of support to the government and this authority, with the aim of advising on mental health policy, assisting in planning and coordination of responses, monitoring the quality of outside technical assistance, and helping to assist with reconstruction to build a sustainable national mental health service capacity and resource mobilization.[56]

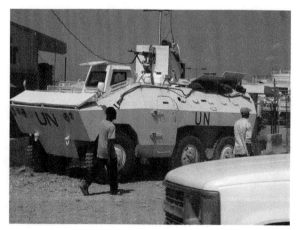

Fig. 5. UN presence (February 2010, G. Raviola). A UN armored vehicle outside a UN compound in Port-au-Prince.

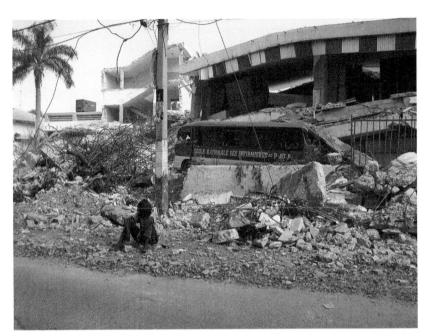

Fig. 6. University hospital (February 2010, G. Raviola). The nursing school at the university hospital in Port-au-Prince collapsed.

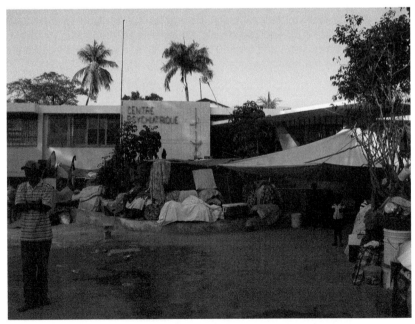

Fig. 7. Psychiatric hospital (February 2010, G. Raviola). The Centre Hospitalier Universitaire de Psychiatrie (University Hospital Center of Psychiatry) Mars and Kline (CHUP/MK), Port-au-Prince, Haiti.

Box 1
IASC, OCHA, and Sphere: coordination of emergency response in disasters

The IASC, created in 1992 by the UN, has served as an interagency forum for coordination, policy development, and decision making involving key UN and non-UN humanitarian partners. The UN Office for the Coordination of Humanitarian Affairs (OCHA) was created in 1998 to assist governments in mobilizing international assistance when the scale of a disaster exceeds national capacity. OCHA manages several tools to facilitate coordination of multiple actors and resources through the UN Cluster approach, a forum of the most experienced relief agencies. Its aim is to strengthen partnerships and ensure more predictability and accountability in international responses to humanitarian emergencies by clarifying the division of labor among organizations and better defining their roles and responsibilities within the key sectors of the response. Initiated in 2000, Sphere describes a set of Minimum Standards to be attained in disaster assistance in each of 5 key sectors: water supply and sanitation; nutrition; food aid; shelter; and health services. Sphere includes indicators for mental and social aspects of health. Questions remain regarding the scientific evidence for particular interventions.

Mental health services

Following the earthquake it was recognized by the Haitian government that mental health had been a neglected area (Alex Larsen, Minister of Health, personal communication, February 2010). The need for mental health services was noted in the MSPP 2010–11 interim health plan.[27] Shortcomings in the educational system for physicians and nurses as well as in the training of specialists were also recognized. Estimates of mental health staffing in the country in 2011 included 194 psychologists (either undergraduate or graduate levels), 82 social workers, 27 psychiatrists (either indigenous or

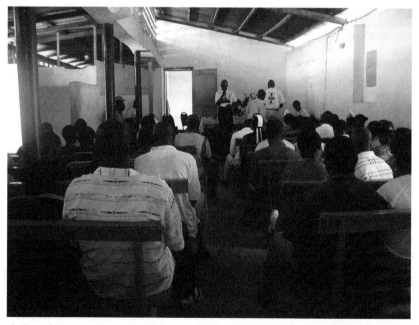

Fig. 8. Zanmi Lasante mourning (February 2010, G. Raviola). A Zanmi Lasante ceremony in Cerca La Source, Haiti. Religious mourning ceremonies were an important post-earthquake intervention to support grieving.

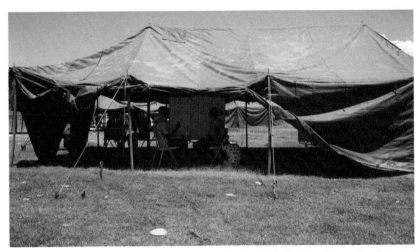

Fig. 9. Zanmi Lasante IDP clinic (February 2010, G. Raviola). A Zanmi Lasante clinic tent in Parc Jean Marie Vincent, Port-au-Prince, Haiti, where a psychologist provides direct clinical services. Nongovernmental organizations delivered clinical services in the IDP settlements.

expatriate), 14 general practitioners trained in provision of mental health care, 3 psychiatric nurses, and 1 neurologist.[14] Of the psychiatrists, the majority were engaged in private practice or NGOs, with the remaining working in the public sector.[14] This analysis is complicated by the fact that a number of NGOs also work to strengthen the public sector. Help-seeking behavior with regard to mental health care has continued to be determined largely by practices existing before the earthquake, with self-referral to a diverse array of traditional and urban healers, and less commonly to biomedical mental health services. The significant influx of foreign clinicians and religious missionaries from a wide array of organizations highlighted the lack of regulation over the safety and quality of interventions, either foreign or local (**Fig. 10**). Broadly, over time services offered by nongovernmental entities included community education and awareness campaigns, psychosocial assistance, mourning, and group support for grief or emerging problems such as cholera, training of physicians and nurses in mental health care, individual psychotherapy and psychopharmacology, and complementary therapies such as acupuncture.[12] Depending on the organization, there existed a range of services and provider types, both local and foreign, across nonspecialist care, social work, psychology, and psychiatry (**Table 1**).

Over 2010 to 2011, through collaboration between MSPP, PAHO, nongovernmental partners, and key partners, there was increased momentum toward articulation of a policy and national strategy for mental health. Planning meetings were organized by the MSPP authority. However, elections with shifts in political leadership, and the shifting of commitments by NGOs, to both Haiti and mental health, have presented challenges in sustaining the process. A working group composed of representatives from MSPP, the xxx psychiatric hospitals, local and international NGOs, and WHO/PAHO was convened through the cluster in the second half of 2010 with the goal of establishing initial steps toward a national policy and plan for mental health. In-country advisory representation of WHO/PAHO to MSPP on mental health was supportive to that process.

Today, however, there remains no mental health plan and policy, and mental health legislation is not yet well defined.[14] Mental health services are not covered for most

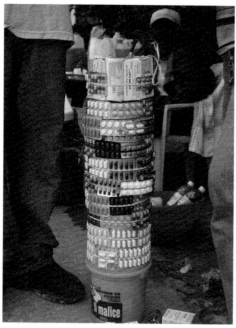

Fig. 10. Street medicine (March 2010, G. Raviola). Street medicines available in Port-au-Prince, Haiti.

Haitians, except for those who can afford insurance systems. Although 30% of the population has access to free psychotropic medication available generally through private sector donations, the cost of 1 day of treatment for antipsychotic and antidepressant medication is prohibitive for a national income average of US$2 per day.[14] Regarding outpatient care, few services are provided, the majority by NGOs.[14] There is no specific outpatient or inpatient care for children and adolescents. Day-treatment facilities or residential services integrated with community psychiatric hospitalization do not exist.

IMPLICATIONS
Coordination and Collaboration: Emergency Response

Postdisaster settings pose substantial challenges for rapid emergency response, including for mental health and psychosocial needs. This is particularly so in contexts of very limited resources, fragmented governance, and lack of pre-event formal mental health infrastructure, as existed in Haiti. Globally a particular challenge has been the coordination of interventions by local and foreign NGOs, groups, and individuals in implementing safe and culturally relevant practices. Regarding mental health, experience has shown the importance of providing culturally and contextually sensitive, integrated, and coordinated interventions informed by qualitative and quantitative assessments of needs, urgency, and resource availability.[57] In Haiti specifically, since the earthquake challenges have been documented broadly in the functioning of humanitarian mechanisms, including: introduction of the UN Cluster process in an exclusive, top-down manner in disregard of local context and existing coordination structures, potentially undermining local ownership and coordination of humanitarian, reconstruction, and development initiatives with Haitian civil society groups; weak

Table 1
Mental health and psychosocial support in Haiti at 8 months

Types of Activities and Implementing Organizations	
MHPSS Activity	Organization
Individual psychological support	ACF, ADRA, AVSI, CW, HI, IMC, MdM-C, MdM-Fr, MdM-Sp, MSF-Bel, MSF-H, MSF-Sp, PIH/ZL, PsF, WV
Group psychological support/counseling	ACF, AVSI, CW, HI, IMC, IOM, MdM-C, MdM-Fr, MdM-Sp, MSF-Bel, MSF-H, MSF-Sp, PIH/ZL, PsF
Psychotropic medications	IMC, MSPP, PIH/ZL
Psychotherapy	ACF, CW, IMC, MSF-Bel, PIH/ZL
Other psychological/psychiatric support	IMC, SI
Case management/social work	IMC, MdM-C, MdM-Fr, MSF-Bel, MSF-H, MSF-Sp, PIH/ZL, PsF
Child-friendly spaces	ACT, ADRA, AVSI, FfH, IMC, IOM, MDM-Fr, PIH/ZL, PiN, PI, StC, SI, TdH, UNICEF
Recreational activities	AVSI, FfH, IMC, IOM, MdM-C, MdM-Fr, PIH/ZL, SI, UNESCO, UNICEF
Including psychosocial consideration in Protection activities	ADRA, IMC, IOM, MdM-Fr, PIH/ZL, PI, PsF, TdH
Facilitating conditions for community mobilization	FfH, MdM-Fr, MdM-Sp, PIH/ZL, PsF, TdH, UNICEF
Strengthening community support and self-help	ADRA, AVSI, FfH, IOM, MdM-C, MdM-Fr, MdM-Sp, MSF-H, PIH/ZL, PsF, RCH, TdH, UNICEF
Vocational training and livelihood assistance	ACF, PIH/ZL
Advocacy	TdH
Providing information to the community	ACF, AVSI, FfH, IOM, MdM-C, MdM-Fr, MdM-Sp, MSF-Bel, MSF-H, PIH/ZL, PsF, TdH, VR
Supporting teachers' psychosocial well-being and training	AVSI, MSF-Bel, PIH/ZL, PI, SI, TdH, UNESCO
Social considerations in nutrition, and WATSAN	ACF, ADRA, AVSI, FfH, IOM, PI, SI, TdH, UNICEF
Other social support	TdH
General activities to support MHPSS	HI, IMC, RCF, IOM, MdM-Sp, MC, PsF, SI, UNICEF, WV

Reporting members: Action Contre la Faim France (ACF), Lutheran World Federation-ACT (ACT), Adventist Development and Relief Agency (ADRA), Ananda Marga Universal Relief Team (AMURT), Association of Volunteers in International Service (AVSI), Christian Blind Mission (CBM), Comité de la Cour des Enfants de Quettstar (COCEQ), Concern Worldwide (CW), Christian Relief Fund (CRF), Food for the Hungry (FfH), Haitian Red Cross/Red Crescent Movement (HRC), Handicap International (HI), International Medical Corps (IMC), International Organization for Migration (IOM), Médecins du Monde Canada (MdM-C), Médecins du Monde France (MdM-Fr), Médecins du Monde Spain (MdM-Sp), Médecins Sans Frontières Belgium (MSF-Bel), Médecins Sans Frontières Holland (MSF-H), Médecins Sans Frontières Spain (MSF-Sp), Médecins Sans Frontières Suisse (MSF-Su), Mercy Corps (MC), Ministère de la Sante Publique et de la Population, Haiti (MSPP), Partners In Health/Zanmi Lasante (PIH/ZL), People in Need (PiN), Plan International (PI), Pharmaciens Sans Frontières Comité International (PsF), Red Cross France (RCF), Red Cross Holland (RCH), Save the Children (StC), Start International (SI), Terres des Hommes (TdH), United Nations Educational, Scientific and Cultural Organization (UNESCO), United Nations Children's Fund (UNICEF), Viva Rio (VR), World Vision (WV).

Abbreviations: MHPSS, Mental Health and Psychosocial Support Network; WATSAN, water and sanitation.

Data from MHPSS Working Group HAITI. Mental health and psychosocial support in Haiti: minimal response matrix and mapping. September, 2010. Available at: http://mhpss.net/wp-content/uploads/group-documents/167/1340873925-haiti-MHPSSMapping-revisedversionSep2010.pdf.

intercluster coordination and predictable leadership regarding multisectoral and cross-cutting issues; and poor communication between the cluster approach and broader humanitarian coordination efforts, with limited emphasis on participatory approaches or accountability toward affected populations.[11,58,59] Given also the profound lack of preexisting medical services, the fragmentation of health care delivery among a large number of NGOs, and the absence of formal mental health services, to some degree ineffective coordination in the planning and delivery of mental health and psychosocial services in the immediate disaster setting would unfortunately be inevitable; this despite the laudable effort to organize activities through the UN Cluster under the leadership of MSPP, also in accordance with the UN IASC guidelines. The guidelines were useful in framing initial action within a pragmatic, do-no-harm, human rights–based approach.[54] Although they emphasize the importance of securing the engagement and participation of local leaders and experts across disciplines, in practice this sometimes did not occur in the Haiti situation, nor was there a template for long-term planning for sustainable services. In the future, better systems are needed for the on-the-ground guidance of emergency mental health and psychosocial response, and facilitation of the transformation of short-term to long-term response.

Coordination and Collaboration: Long-Term Service Planning

Such complexity and challenge has tended to only aggravate the tendency to approach postdisaster needs in an episodic fashion with deployment of external resources, rather than as an opportunity to build local capacity and purposefully lay the groundwork for sustained delivery with attention to building the foundation for services and long-term development. The earthquake also exposed a public-sector mental health system in disrepair.[60,61] Several efforts have sought to support more sustained capacity in the country over time, building on and within accepted primary health care structures. Through the integration of plural local belief systems, pragmatic use of existing and emerging evidence-based practices, and adaptation of existing primary care and community-based care models, there is opportunity to attempt to develop continua of care incorporating culturally relevant psychoeducation for the wider community, psychosocial support for those in distress, and a range of appropriate clinical services for the more severely affected and mentally ill.[62–64] One example of such an effort has been undertaken by Partners In Health/Zanmi Lasante (PIH/ZL).[12] The presence of the PIH/ZL health care system in Haiti over the past 25 years, serving approximately 1.2 million people in Haiti's Central Plateau and Artibonite Valley and providing hospital and community health worker-based care for HIV and tuberculosis, has offered a unique platform that could be a foundation on which to build a similar integrated system of mental health care. ZL had taken steps before the earthquake to provide psychosocial services to certain high-need medical populations, and thus had in place several social workers and bachelor's-level psychologists who formed the base on which to mount a more comprehensive, integrative community-based strategy with limited resources. ZL identified and adopted a specific, evidence-supported planning and implementation framework to guide its efforts, currently under way and supported by Grand Challenges Canada, for scaled integrated mental health care throughout its system to take advantage of that foundation for long-term capacity in the context of a short-term disaster response.[64] It is hoped that the use of such deliberate and structured efforts, among others, can in the future collectively support the establishment of a decentralized, community-based system led by the government across Haiti's 10 departments. Doing so will require providers and actors to engage community health centers and community health workers, encourage associations of users and families, and support mental health services offered at district hospitals and at a small number of higher-quality psychiatric facilities in order to support and anchor a community-based foundation. A commitment to establishing a national policy and strategic plan for mental health will also need to be sustained, by both the government and other partners.

ACKNOWLEDGMENTS

The authors are grateful to Kate Boyd, MPH, Shin Daimyo, MPH, Paul Farmer, MD, PhD, and Claire-Cecille Pierre, MD, for their critical review and comments.

REFERENCES

1. Farmer P. The uses of Haiti. Monroe (ME): Common Courage Press; 2006. p. 65–74.
2. Masters J. Wunderground.com. Hurricanes and Haiti: a tragic history. Available at: http://www.wunderground.com/resources/education/haiti.asp. Accessed December 15, 2012.
3. WHO/PAHO. Culture and mental health in Haiti: a literature review. Geneva (Switzerland): WHO; 2010.
4. Corten A. Diabolisation et Mai Politique. Haïti: misère, religion et politique. Montreal (Canada): les Editions CIDIHCA; 2000.
5. Hurbon L. La conjunction des imaginaires européen et africain autour du Vodou. In: Hainard J, Mathez P, Schinz O, editors. Vodou. Geneva (Switzerland): Infolio, Musee d'ethnographie de Geneve; 2008. p. 105–12.
6. Brodwin PE. Guardian angels and dirty spirits: the moral basis of healing power in rural Haiti. In: Nichter M, editor. Anthropological approaches to the study of ethnomedicine. Langhorne (PA): Gordon & Breach; 1992.
7. Brodwin PE. Medicine and morality in Haiti: the contest for healing power. New York: Cambridge University Press; 1996.
8. Globalsecurity.org. Haiti—introduction. Available at: http://www.globalsecurity.org/military/world/haiti/intro.htm. Accessed December 15, 2012.
9. Métraux A. Le Vaudou Haïtien. Paris: Gallimard; 1958.
10. Sterlin C. Pour une approche interculturelle du concept de santé. In: Ruptures, revue transdisciplinaire en santé 2006;77(1):112–21.
11. Binder A, Grünewald F. Haiti: IASC cluster approach evaluation, 2nd phase country study, April 2010. Groupe Urgence Réhabilitation Dévelopment and Global Public Policy Institute. p. 7.
12. Raviola G, Eustache E, Oswald C, et al. Mental health response in the aftermath of the 2010 Haiti earthquake: a case study for long-term solutions. Harv Rev Psychiatry 2012;20(1):68–77.
13. CIA World Factbook. Available at: https://www.cia.gov/library/publications/the-world-factbook/geos/ha.html. Accessed December 15, 2012.
14. WHO. Le système de santé mentale en Haïti: rapport d'évaluation du système de Santé mentale en Haïti a l'aide de l'instrument d'evaluation conçu par L'Organization Mondiale de la Santé Mentale (OMS). Ministère de la Santé Publique et de la. Population, Organisation Mondiale de la Santé, Organisation Panaméricaine de la Santé. 2011.
15. The majority of households in Haiti do not have access to electricity, particularly in rural areas. Trading Economics. Available at: www.tradingeconomics.com/haiti/access-to-electricity-percent-of-population-wb-data.html. Accessed July 19, 2013.

16. Özden C. Brain Drain in Latin America. Development Research Group. The World Bank; 2005. p. 3.
17. Kristoff M, Panarelli L. Haiti: a republic of NGOs? United States Institute of Peace Brief; April 26, 2010. p. 1–3.
18. Doyle M. BBC: US urged to stop Haiti rice subsidies. October 4, 2010. Available at: http://www.bbc.co.uk/news/world-latin-america-11472874. Accessed December 15, 2012.
19. Pan American Health Organization. Haiti: Profile of the Health Services System. Second edition, July 2003. p. 2.
20. Miller NL. Haitian ethnomedical systems and biomedical practitioners: directions for clinicians. J Transcult Nurs 2000;11(3):204–11.
21. Deren M. Divine horsemen: the living gods of Haiti. Documentext. New Paltz (NY): MacPherson; 1983.
22. Sterlin C. Pour une approche interculturelle du concept de santé. Ruptures, revue transdisciplinaire en santé 2006;11(1):112–21.
23. Gopaul-McNicol S, Benjamin-Dartigue D, Francois M. Working with Haitian Canadian families. Int J Adv Couns 1998;20:231–42.
24. Desrosiers A, St Fleurose S. Treating Haitian patients: key cultural aspects. Am J Psychother 2002;56(4):508–21.
25. Farmer P. The birth of the Klinik: a cultural history of Haitian professional psychiatry. In: Gaines A, editor. Ethnopsychiatry. Albany (NY): SUNY; 1992. p. 251–72.
26. Mars LP. Paranoïa et mythomanie en Haïti. 1937.
27. Ministère de la Santé Publique et de la Population. Plan Interimaire Du Sectuer Santé, Avril 2010–Septembre 2011. Mars 2010. p. 6.
28. OCHA. Annual plan and budget. Responding in a Changing World. 2011:57.
29. Office of the Special Envoy for Haiti. Available at: http://www.haitispecialenvoy.org/relief-and-recovery/key-statistics/. Accessed December 15, 2012.
30. Disaster Emergency Committee. Available at: http://www.dec.org.uk/haiti-earthquake-facts-and-figures. Accessed December 15, 2012.
31. Hendriksen RS, Price LB, Schupp JM, et al. Population genetics of *Vibrio cholerae* from Nepal in 2010: evidence on the origin of the Haitian outbreak. MBio 2011;2(4):e00157. p. 11.
32. Centers for Disease Control and Prevention. Available at: http://www.cdc.gov/haiticholera/haiti_cholera.htm. Accessed December 15, 2012.
33. Wise C. Fighting cholera, a dose at a time. PBS. Available at: http://www.pbs.org/newshour/rundown/2012/12/fighting-cholera-in-haiti-one-dose-at-a-time.html. Accessed December 15, 2012.
34. Landau E. In Haiti, mental aftershocks could be far-reaching. CNN. January 19, 2010. Available at: http://www.cnn.com/2010/HEALTH/01/15/haiti.mental.psychological.effects/index.html. Accessed December 15, 2012.
35. Kaplan A. Haiti earthquake: mental health needs are emerging. Psychiatric Times 2010.
36. Smith M. Psychiatrists predict Haitians face long-term mental health issues. Voice of America News 2010.
37. Bajak F. Mental health in Haiti: nation copes with trauma. Huffington Post 2010.
38. Ben-Ezra M, Shrira A, Palgi Y. The hidden face of Haiti's tragedy. Science 2010; 327:1325.
39. PBS Newshour. In Haiti, mental health still a concern for many quake survivors. July 15, 2010. Available at: http://www.pbs.org/newshour/bb/latin_america/july-dec10/haiti_07-15.html. Accessed December 15, 2012.
40. OCHA. Humanitarian bulletin. March 10-25, 2011. p. 2–3.

41. Haiti Advocacy Working Group. Health Challenges in Haiti. 2010. p. 3–4.
42. UNICEF. Children in Haiti. One year after: the long road from relief to recovery. 2011. p. 4–19.
43. UNICEF. Humanitarian action report mid-year review: partnering for children in emergencies. 2010. p. 157–60.
44. Institute for Justice and Democracy in Haiti, Trans Africa Forum, MADRE, University of Minnesota Law School, University of Virginia School of Law. Our bodies are still trembling: Haitian women's fight against rape. 2010. p. 4–30.
45. Nicholas G, DeSilva A, Prater K, et al. Empathic family stress as a sign of family connectedness in Haitian immigrants. Fam Process 2009;48(1):135–50.
46. Montpetit J. Depression, psychological trauma in Canada's Haitian community year after quake. The Canadian Press; 2011.
47. Cox L. Haiti relief workers risk their minds. ABC News 2010.
48. Carson N, Cook BL, Alegria M. Determinants of mental health treatment among Haitian, African American, and White Youth in community health centers. J Health Care Poor Underserved 2010;21:32–48.
49. Stige SH, Sveaass N. Psychologist. Living in exile when disaster strikes at home. Torture 2010;20(2):76–91.
50. Muller D. Haiti: a piece of my mind. JAMA 2011;305(5):447–8.
51. OCHA. Haiti: one year later. Available at: http://www.unocha.org/issues-in-depth/haiti-one-year-later. Accessed December 15, 2012.
52. OCHA. Haiti—population movements out of Port-au-Prince as of 28 January 2010. Available at: http://reliefweb.int/map/haiti/haiti-population-movements-out-port-au-prince-28-january-2010. Accessed December 15, 2012.
53. World Health Organization. Humanitarian action: health cluster guide. Available at: http://www.who.int/hac/global_health_cluster/guide/en/index.html. Accessed December 15, 2012.
54. Inter-Agency Standing Committee (IASC). IASC guidelines on mental health and psychosocial support in emergency settings. Geneva (Switzerland): IASC; 2007.
55. Jones L. Mental health in disaster settings: new humanitarian guidelines include the needs of people with severe mental disorders. Br Med J 2007;335:679–80.
56. Saxena S, van Ommeren M, Saraceno B. Mental health assistance to populations affected by disasters: World Health Organization's role. Int Rev Psychiatry 2006;18(3):199–204.
57. Ghodse H, Galea S. Tsunami: understanding mental health consequences and the unprecedented response. Int Rev Psychiatry 2006;18(3):289–97.
58. Refugees International. Field Report, Haiti: from the ground up. March 2, 2010. p. 1–4.
59. Moszynski P. International response risks undermining Haiti's health system, warns relief agency. Br Med J 2011;342:d182.
60. Sontag S. In Haiti, mental health system is in collapse. New York Times 2010.
61. Ellingwood K. Haitians' deep aftershocks. Los Angeles Times 2010.
62. Jones LM, Ghani1 HA, Mohanraj A, et al. Crisis into opportunity: setting up community mental health services in post-tsunami Aceh. Asia Pac J Public Health 2007;19(Special issue):60–8.
63. Belkin G, Unützer J, Kessler R, et al. Scaling up for the "bottom billion": 5 × 5 implementation of community mental health care in low-income regions. Psychiatr Serv 2011;62(12):1494–502.
64. Grand Challenges Canada. Our grantees: Global Mental Health (Round 1). Available at: http://www.grandchallenges.ca/globalmentalhealth-grantees-EN/. Accessed July 10, 2013.

Community Engagement in Disaster Preparedness and Recovery

A Tale of Two Cities – Los Angeles and New Orleans

Kenneth B. Wells, MD, MPH[a,b,c,]*,
Benjamin F. Springgate, MD, MPH[c], Elizabeth Lizaola, MPH[a],
Felica Jones[d], Alonzo Plough, PhD, MPH[e]

KEYWORDS

- Disasters • Disaster response • Community engagement • Community health
- Behavioral health

KEY POINTS

- Awareness of the impact of disasters globally on mental health is increasing.
- Known difficulties in preparing communities for disasters and a lack of focus on relationship building and organizational capacity in preparedness and response have led to a greater policy focus on community resiliency as a key public health approach to disaster response.
- This perspective emphasizes relationships, trust, and engagement as core competencies for disaster preparedness and response/recovery.
- Our approach has a specific focus on behavioral health and relationship building across diverse sectors and stakeholders concerned with underresourced communities.

[a] Center for Health Services and Society, Semel Institute for Neuroscience and Human Behavior, University of California, Los Angeles, 10920 Wilshire Boulevard, Suite 300, Los Angeles, CA 90024, USA; [b] Department of Health Policy and Management, Jonathan and Karin Fielding School of Public Health and Department of Psychiatry and Biobehavioral Sciences, David Geffen School of Medicine, University of California, Los Angeles, 760 Westwood Plaza, Los Angeles, CA 90024, USA; [c] RAND Health, RAND Corporation, 1776 Main Street, Santa Monica, CA 90401, USA; [d] Healthy African American Families, 4305 Degnan Boulevard, Los Angeles, CA 90008, USA; [e] Los Angeles County Department of Public Health, Emergency Preparedness and Response, 500 W. Temple Street, Los Angeles, CA 90012, USA
* Corresponding author.
E-mail address: kwells@mednet.ucla.edu

Psychiatr Clin N Am 36 (2013) 451–466
http://dx.doi.org/10.1016/j.psc.2013.05.002
0193-953X/13/$ – see front matter © 2013 Elsevier Inc. All rights reserved.

BACKGROUND

Recent disasters such as Katrina/Gulf storms, the September 11 terrorist attacks, and Superstorm Sandy have increased awareness among policy makers, providers, and the public concerning long-term health risks, including psychological distress, from disaster exposure and the key role that first responders, nurses, other medical and emergency response staff, and volunteers, play in mitigating risks early by helping to assure safety, services linkage, and support for physical, mental, and social well-being. Large-scale disasters disrupt physical, social, and communication infrastructures and diminish coping resources and social supports[1–3] and pose both temporary and long-term threats to physical and psychological health.[4] One of the key barriers to recovery among vulnerable populations is high risk of mental distress and disorders[4,5] that interfere with effective help-seeking and timely evacuation and increase risk for other long-term health outcomes.[6,7] A subset of affected people develop new disorders and chronic illness and impairment.[8,9] Public health threats such as infectious disease outbreaks and radiation exposure also threaten health security and create often disproportionate distress in vulnerable groups in underresourced communities.[10–12]

All persons exposed to disasters are vulnerable, but subgroups including children[12] and underresourced ethnic minority communities[10–12] are at high risk for poor outcomes. Underresourced communities such as urban communities of color are at higher risk for poorer health outcomes owing to preexisting disparities in health, access to services, and environmental risk factors.[1,13,14] They also face disparities in disaster response time and outcomes.[15,16] Disasters generate multiple stressors that can trigger ongoing psychological distress in such vulnerable groups,[17] as observed post-Katrina.[6,18,19] Given that disasters are unexpected and local resources are often overwhelmed, response is facilitated by first responders from government agencies and volunteer responders from community-based agencies including Volunteer Organizations Active in Disasters. First responders also include nurses and other medical staff from public health and medical clinics and hospitals, emergency response agencies, schools, and volunteers of agencies such as faith-based groups and neighborhood associations. Responders have diverse roles in preparedness (outreach, training), response (assessment, services, referral), and recovery (services rebuilding and coordination). All first responders are also at high risk for psychological distress and unmet need.[20]

To address the broader social and environmental factors that may affect outcomes of disaster preparedness, response, and longer-term recovery efforts, Community Disaster Resilience (CDR) has emerged as recent national policy priority.[21,22] CDR follows a community systems model[23] that emphasizes communication, partnership and activating networks around disaster-response goals, and community engagement[24,25] and improved provider communication with underserved populations.[26,27] However, there has been no operational definition of CDR or model demonstration of how best to apply these principles in practice in vulnerable communities. Building capacity for CDR requires an approach suitable to integrating and coordinating the perspectives and skills of diverse stakeholders, including historically vulnerable groups, first responders, and experts in evidence-based approaches to improving outcomes, including for mental health consequences of disasters. Because Community-Based Participatory Research (CBPR) is recommended for both program development and research with vulnerable groups,[28–36] it offers one approach to develop and operationalize CDR.

Community-Partnered Participatory Research (CPPR)[37,38] is a manualized form of CBPR that is suitable for this purpose as it promotes equal power and authority of diverse community and academic partners to develop and evaluate programs while building scientific and community capacity for using findings and products.[37] CPPR promotes two-way knowledge exchange across diverse stakeholders through a community engagement paradigm. We use the term "community" to refer to persons who work, share recreation, or live in a given area. Community engagement refers to values, strategies, and actions that support authentic partnerships, including mutual respect and inclusive participation, power sharing and equity, and flexibility in goals, methods, and timeframes to fit priorities and capacities of communities.[28,37] The CPPR approach is asset-based and designed to build community capacity while developing knowledge for scientific and community benefit. A key strategy is identifying the "win-win" or fit of goals across stakeholders. A CPPR initiative involves forming a partnered Council, identifying experts to support the work and community forums for broad input.[39] CPPR unfolds in 3 stages: Vision (planning), Valley (work), and Victory (products, dissemination) and supports evaluation within a participatory approach.[37,38]

During the past 10 years, we have developed this framework and approach to applying CPPR to address mental health outcome disparities in underresourced communities of color in Los Angeles and mental health recovery post-disaster in New Orleans. Our work across these 2 areas has evolved in stages enabling us to apply lessons learned across projects and share resources across communities iteratively. The signature projects for the evolution of our approach are Witness for Wellness/ Community Partners in Care (CPIC) in Los Angeles,[39–42] the REACH NOLA Mental Health Infrastructure and Training (MHIT) Program for post-Katrina disaster recovery[43] in New Orleans, and the Los Angeles County Community Disaster Resilience (LACCDR) initiative. All projects were supported in part by the Partnered Research Center (PRC) for Quality Care, which aims to conduct research following a CPPR approach to improve mental health outcomes.[44] Overall, the Center follows a learning community model to promote community-engaged approaches to address mental health disparities and to develop a community resilience approach to disaster preparedness and response (**Fig. 1**).

In the framework, community engagement promoting equal decision making through two-way knowledge exchange is combined with policy support to promote

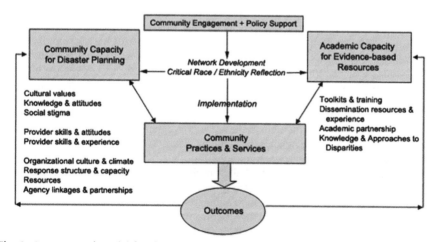

Fig. 1. A conceptual model for the community engagement approach to disaster response, including for mental health that has emerged from the "tale of 2 cities."

network development and integration of community and academic/clinical and public health perspectives and to generate programs that are implemented and evaluated to build CDR or improve mental health outcomes. A key component of the development of networks, policy, and implementation, however, is attention to the salience of race and ethnicity, a process of leadership reflection emerging from critical race theory.[45,46] This helps assure that programs developed and their implementation will be equitable from a social justice perspective. The program implementation in services lead to outcomes that are also determined in partnership; and the results of the evaluation are used in a feedback loop to build community and academic capacity and inform policymakers to provide further support for effective and equitable programs for disaster planning. Such a community-learning framework integrates multiple theories, such as social learning, expert opinion, and organizational learning and quality improvement theory, within an overall socioecological framework.

"TALE OF 2 CITIES" CASE STUDY

The application of the CPPR model to mental health began with the Witness for Wellness (W4W) project, which paved the way for the model to be applied successfully in subsequent programs. This project was designed to address the issue of depression and to begin exploring ways of overcoming the stigma associated with it.[39,47–50] Although not implemented in a post-disaster context, W4W was designed and implemented in the resource-poor, urban setting of South Los Angeles. The project was initiated through a planning process that presented to nearly 500 community representatives information on both community-based approaches to address depression and evidence from research studies of collaborative care and other treatment models for depression in low-income minority communities.[39] Next, a large planning process[48] using multistakeholder sharing and consensus methods led to the formulation of 3 community-academic co-led working groups: (1) Talking Wellness addressed social stigma of depression and worked to identify culturally appropriate ways of increasing the dialogue in South Los Angeles about the salience of depression as an issue for community action[47]; (2) Building Wellness responded to concerns about scarcity of health care providers in Los Angeles by developing approaches to support screening and case management for depressed clients through social services settings,[50] using as a starting point the quality improvement toolkits from the Partners in Care study[51]; and (3) Supporting Wellness developed strategies to bring the issue of depression to the attention of policy makers and advocate for the support of vulnerable communities to address depression.[49] The project led to several innovations locally such as use of the arts to engage the community to build collective efficacy to address depression.[52] A regular feature of this project was reflection on equity and the salience of race and ethnicity within the project leadership. As one example, the lead community PI was an African American woman and the lead academic PI a Caucasian man. Their partnership included many discussions of equalizing power. Community members, after initially wondering about the appropriateness of having a Caucasian academic lead, became very supportive after engaging in an open discussion of concerns about the potential for racism and a history of white supremacy as a threat to the community. The strong partnership of academic and community leaders, which grew over time, helped to achieve a balance that was often commented on by other leaders and community members at meetings.[38,53] This project had a high representation of unaffiliated community members with high levels of social and/or health needs in leadership and membership positions, who worked regularly with academic leaders and system/clinical leaders from the community. To achieve this goal, the project had a very strong focus on diversity, trust building, development of common language and concepts, and transparency, and most conflicts arising during the course of this project were over these issues rather than the content of program planning.[37]

Overall, the W4W initiative illustrated that addressing mental health challenges such as depression in vulnerable communities through a community engagement approach, can be a "win-win". Community members and agencies gained knowledge of and confidence in addressing depression and familiarity with evidence-based approaches, whereas researchers and community members worked together on community and academic products concerning mental health. This project gave us confidence in the ability of clinicians and nonclinicians, both community and academic, to work together to plan large-scale mental health improvement initiatives in underresourced communities. Policymakers were also directly involved in the workgroups, which helped develop opportunities to align community goals with policy opportunities, such as representing community perspectives in large stakeholder processes in Los Angeles County.[49]

Although large-scale implementation of the resources developed in the W4W initiative had not yet occurred in Los Angeles, the partnership model and specific tools were developed sufficiently to be helpful as resources to the REACH NOLA MHIT Program, a Red Cross–funded initiative to promote mental health recovery post-Katrina in New Orleans. This initiative's relationship with the PRC at University of California, Los Angeles/Research and Development (RAND) developed because the PRC Center Director was the main mentor for a Robert Wood Johnson Foundation Clinical Scholar at UCLA from New Orleans; at the time, the RWJF program had recently expanded to have a major focus on community engagement as a skill for clinician investigators.[54] In this context, a new collaboration formed to develop an approach to promote mental health recovery after hurricanes Katrina and Rita.

Post-Katrina New Orleans was an area in great need of mental health services, but with minimal access to such care because of damage to much of the traditional health care infrastructure of the city.[1–4,43] The MHIT initiative aimed to address this unmet need and build capacity by activating partnerships among academic institutions including RAND, UCLA, and Tulane and community agencies including faith-based organizations, clinics and health centers, and social services agencies. MHIT embraced CPPR principles such as power and resource sharing, co-planning of activities by community and academic investigators, and formal recognition of community input. For example, as in the W4W initiative, MHIT was led by a steering council comprising community and academic partners to help prioritize project goals and activities. The Council also ensured that specific arrangements were in place to support community and academic partners equally with regards to funding and decision making; this helped to build capacity as did the experience gained by community and academic partners from contributing to all program phases from inception, relating to funders, implementation, assessment, and dissemination of products or results.

MHIT grew out of an initial 1-year post-storm assessment of need for services in New Orleans, which identified high unmet need for mental health services as a key recovery issue.[43] To address those needs, MHIT integrated prior evidence-based approaches to improving quality of care and outcomes for depression at a systems level: Partners in Care,[51] We Care,[55] and IMPACT.[56] However, because of the lack of stable health care infrastructure even 1-year post-Katrina and trust issues among the communities most heavily affected by the disaster, the CPPR model as developed in the W4W initiative helped to inform the overall approach to MHIT. MHIT, however, was funded specifically to build services capacity and thus offered an opportunity to implement the lessons from W4W at some scale. Using a community engagement approach modified for the unique, post-storm environment in New Orleans, MHIT provided training in Cognitive Behavioral Therapy for depression; medication management; team management of depression; and case management skills, including screening for depression and other health and life difficulties, behavioral activation and problem solving, outcomes tracking, and other relevant skills. A significant accomplishment of MHIT was the development of a community health worker/outreach worker manual to support screening, education, outcomes tracking, referral, and the basics of behavioral activation and problem solving at a much broader scale.[57] MHIT implemented 75 trainings over 2 years involving more than 400 providers in community-based agencies and potentially reached more than 110,000 community members with improvements in outreach, screening, assessment, and treatment and/or case management or support for depression and trauma-related symptoms.[43] Achieving capacity building at this scale also required developing relationships with local and state-level policy makers as well as clinicians and community leaders. In addition, this project brought awareness that the providers being trained oftentimes had the same issues in terms of post-disaster consequences for mental health as the clients they were serving. The repeated exposure through services provision to others in distress posed challenges to providers who themselves were at risk for distress post-trauma. In response, we also developed an approach to provider self-care as a routine part of trainings, using alternative therapies and simple strategies such as training in behavioral activation to assist coping strategies. Like the W4W initiative, this services demonstration also had strong representation of community members, although many held a leadership role, whether heading a neighborhood association or providing volunteer or professional case management services. However, in the context of recovery from a disaster, most participants were simultaneously serving several roles, such as being a provider or staff member while also being a community member directly affected by the disaster. For this reason, the project was designed to be flexible in expectations as people participated or withdrew due to these different roles and needs.

This substantial experience in implementation of evidence-based or informed services delivery strategies for depression in New Orleans were brought back to Los Angeles and incorporated into the next-generation study after W4W, CPIC.[37,40–42] CPIC was the main partnered scientific goal that emerged from W4W, which was to determine the unique added value of community capacity building under a CPPR model over and above more standard, individual agency training to address depression. CPIC was a randomized trial, itself conducted under CPPR principles and structure, in which nearly 100 programs in Los Angeles providing primary care/ public health, mental health, substance abuse, or social services, as well as other community-based agencies such as faith-based, senior centers, exercise clubs, or hair salons were randomized to one of 2 models of implementing collaborative care for depression: (1) individual agency assistance through webinars and site visits or (2) a period of collaborative planning across all assigned agencies to fit the partnered training plan to the needs and strengths of the community. Outcomes were then tracked for more than a year at both provider/agency and client levels; results are still pending. The project is being conducted in both South Los Angeles, the site for the W4W study, and Hollywood-Metropolitan Los Angeles. Both communities have substantial representation of Latinos and African Americans. The wide range of programs represented in this study were a result of community input, suggesting that this was the range of programs relevant to persons with depression living in the community[40]; and this range was similar to that of programs participating in trainings in the New Orleans MHIT project. Although MHIT did not have a strong outcomes research component, as it was not a research study but a services project, the CPIC study did and was designed as a randomized trial.

To support this range of agencies in identifying components of collaborative care relevant to their scope, the authors used their extensive implementation experience in New Orleans, and the resources developed there such as the Health Worker manual, to inform further adaptations for CPIC. This was particularly appropriate because issues of cultural competence and trust were salient in the Los Angeles and New Orleans environments and although not suffering the consequences of a major disaster, the Los Angeles communities faced many highly stressful issues common in underresourced urban communities of color. In addition, because CPIC providers often lived in the same communities and faced many of the same stresses as their clients, the authors used the provider self-care strategies developed in MHIT and faced similar issues in terms of participants serving multiple roles that needed acknowledgment and accommodation in the process and structure. In CPIC, much of what was new above and beyond the adaptations of the collaborative care models from prior projects was the extensive development of a community-partnered approach to designing and conducting a group-randomized trial; this had not been a component of W4W or MHIT. This experience in community engagement in designing a randomized trial combined with the mental health recovery work in New Orleans led to an opportunity to address disaster preparedness from a community resiliency perspective in the LACCDR initiative.

LACCDR has developed a CDR approach to disaster preparedness using the CPPR model in Los Angeles and like CPIC is following the approach of a participatory public health trial.[58–61] Like W4W, MHIT, and CPIC, LACCDR is led by a steering council, which developed 3 workgroups in its first year to engage stakeholders and identify priorities for building resilient communities. Key stakeholders include first responders, neighborhood watch members, and representatives from faith-based organizations, the business community, and representatives of vulnerable populations. The community engagement approach to developing the LACCDR design is described elsewhere.[59] One key difference between the prior CPPR-informed efforts described earlier and LACCDR is that LACCDR grew out of the initiative of public health policymakers, so the policy support is present from the outset.

LACCDR is designed to explore how to implement a community resiliency approach to disaster preparedness overall and to compare the results for partnerships and community preparedness from a state-of-the art, traditional individual/family preparedness initiative with a broad community resilience initiative in comparable communities. As a preparedness project led by the public health department, LACCDR has a strong focus on responder agencies and their staff and volunteers, who work closely with diverse communities to achieve CDR goals. These goals include improved organizational relationships, salient connections to community leaders and members, and communication strategies to improve access to information and resources. For the purposes of this article, LACCDR represents the next step in the cycle of projects focusing on community engagement for improving mental health and/or disaster response. Although LACCDR does not have a primary mental health focus, it includes a focus on personal and organizational relationships as part of community resilience. In addition, provision of psychological first aid[20] is one core component of the community resiliency toolkits being developed for the pilot demonstration.

LACCDR is also using the CPPR model and some of its adaptation for the community engagement intervention from CPIC to inform its community resiliency intervention model. As an initiative instituted by a policy and services agency, LACCDR has had somewhat less focus on inclusion of unaffiliated community members or those in need of services as participants to date. However, some workgroup leaders are from community-based organizations such as churches or community clinics as well as from advocacy organizations for underresourced communities and special populations.

IMPLICATIONS AND LESSONS LEARNED

Our "tale of 2 cities" has led to many lessons learned concerning the feasibility of a community learning approach to mental health issues in general and to disaster response in particular, with implications for communities, policymakers, and clinicians. Because of the integrated, partnership approach that has evolved iteratively over time, those lessons have emerged from the perspective of diverse stakeholders interacting with each other (**Table 1**).

Mental health as a concern: the authors' experience suggests that although many agree that mental health is a key issue both in general and after disasters and in planning for disasters, working with community is critical to defining the issue and identifying the appropriate language to use in uncovering what mental health and psychological issues mean in community. In some communities affected by disaster, the notion of mental health as an issue (current or future) may be unexpected or even at times denied as a reality. In part this may be because of other pressing and immediate issues, such as housing crises, schools that were destroyed, or levees that failed. As a result, it may require deliberate investigation with affected community members to identify that mental health is (or is not) a significant issue for the population at that time. Further, it may require looking beyond words to behaviors and interactions together.

Trust and capacity issues: there can be substantial insider-outsider dynamics following some disasters that may complicate trust concerns in attempting to build capacity for or provide mental health services. Key to the public approach is early engagement with vulnerable communities before a disaster to collaboratively build a common understanding of the challenges, define the problems, and build capacities to improve resilience. Many people in more normal circumstances are already reluctant to discuss mental health owing to stigma. Discussing research or even health care in community settings even in a nondisaster situation can be fraught with concerns about unequal power dynamics, histories of abuse, and other legitimate concerns, particularly in low-income communities and communities of color. The imposition of a disaster on top of those usual strains may magnify the sense of disparity regarding who is really part of the community and who is an outsider.

Efforts to build trust can overcome those issues, but the sacrifice and investment of time is not necessarily commonplace in disaster response, which is why trust must be built before a disaster. The Federal Emergency Management Agency whole community planning strategy is to incorporate predisaster collaboration between responders and community residents.[21] It may be simpler for a responder agency to provide funding to local agencies to ensure that some services are delivered, as funding agencies may prefer organizations with a solid financial track record, but then the opportunity to build capacity among the most affected agencies that are trusted among the most impacted populations can be lost. Depending on the disaster, this may be hard to come by post-disaster, and approaches are needed to work directly with community-based organizations working in low-income settings. One approach that the authors used post-Katrina in New Orleans was to partner with some medium to larger size agencies and also use a nonprofit research firm (RAND) to partner in managing accountability for smaller agencies.

Research and evaluation: in disaster research, relatively few people living in disaster-affected communities want to spend time being counted so that lessons can be learned and applied to inform future circumstances. There are substantial efforts to engage post-disaster communities in research, but not all have been successful in recruiting participants.[62] Additionally, different communities will prioritize hazards differently and agencies must be responsive to this dynamic. We have learned in the CPIC study and in MHIT that partnered approaches can help overcome these issues, but in the context of programs that built real-time capacity for addressing needs through trainings at scale and with substantial investment of resources in community partners through a co-led enterprise; this requires additional effort and expertise that are uncommon to date. In the future, such efforts will become more common given the new policy directive at FEMA and CDC.

Provider/clinician development issues: the authors found it feasible to engage large numbers of providers in diverse organizations in capacity building for evidence-based collaborative care for depression in MHIT and CPIC. Both of these projects made substantial adjustments to prior research-based implementation strategies, such as simplifying language or tailoring specific components to the actual work scope of a given provider or program. The main modification needed for the disaster and/or underresourced community context was adding provision of support for provider self-care as many of the providers faced similar stresses to their clients, identified with them, or had actually survived the same disaster. Thus, part of the provider development and capacity building issues to address mental health are to anticipate this need. The authors also determined across projects that providers in community-based settings can make excellent training partners to academic experts in leading community trainings. They understand the local context and needs of providers in similar agencies, increasing the relevance of trainings and fit to community assets and capacities. However, the success of capacity building was also directly tied to efforts to maintain culturally competent trainings and services, which took considerable time beyond the usual trainings in evidence-based practice to develop and maintain. From LACCDR, we have learned that tools and capacity-building activities must have real time as well as disaster utility.

Community transparency and leadership: a signature feature of all of these projects was attention to what is referred to in CPPR as transparency, or finding a community language, to arrive at common meanings for concepts, products, and other outcomes such as toolkits or evaluation findings. Given histories of distrust and stressful circumstances in underresourced communities for the consequences of disasters, the sustained effort to communicate important concepts, needs, and approaches and to reach agreements on how best to move forward together were crucial to collaborating in trainings and services delivery. The commitment to transparency might be viewed as at the heart of the co-leadership that emerged in all the projects. Consistently, strong community leaders emerged who led the charge for attending to mental health issues and often became leaders more broadly as a result. This leadership development in the community over sensitive matters such as mental health and depression was one of the striking developments across projects. In this respect, the projects outlined earlier were about much more than developing an approach to disaster or mental health. They were more like a demonstration of the broader principle of the value of developing human capital in diverse forms to address important mental health and community resilience needs. Each of the projects faced a somewhat different course of development regarding community leadership and participation of more "grass

Table 1
Community engagement (CE) issues and lessons learned

CE Issue	Strategy	Challenge	Lesson Learned
Joint leadership	Include community and academic members in all meetings	Members with demanding schedules may not always be available	Embrace the "on the bus, off the bus" model, which recognizes that members can participate as feasible and welcome inclusive participation to sustain project activities
LACCDR: strong focus on first responders	Recruit volunteer first responders	First responders are accustomed to top down approach vs bottom up approach applied in CE projects	Pair first responders from government agencies to operate under hierarchical structures with volunteer responders to balance perspectives
Shared decision making	Executive Steering Council of community and academic members	Community and academic representation may not be equal	Diversify ways of giving input for decisions (e-mail, phone participation; proxy votes) or as needed delay until fuller input is obtained, out of respect for the partnership
CPIC: diverse leadership	Community leaders support each other	Academic leaders may tend to dominate	Pair academic leaders with multiple community co-leads who balance/spell each other
Resource sharing	Provide subawards or consultant payments to partners	Tensions may arise due to perceived inequity in distribution of funds	Transparent budget review, pro-active planning to balance resources and communicate goals to funders
MHIT: provide resources to enable community participation	Subawards and consultant payments to partners	Learning curve for smaller agencies in managing funds and complying with policy	Designate an experienced agency to manage and distribute funds among smaller community-based organizations.
Create shared vision	CE activity (similar to an icebreaker)	Find activities that build relationships while supporting mission and are culturally appropriate.	The most effective CE activities are symbolic of project aims, encourage people to think creatively and get people out of their seats and are jointly led.

All projects: CE exercise	Brief activity that gets people thinking as a group	Academics may initially resist nontraditional meeting activity	Have project leaders/investigators lead the CE exercise to level the playing field and help meeting participants to be engaged
Trust	Identify "win-wins" to demonstrate that community and academic goals are equally valued	May require modification of initial project aims	Training resources that combine scientific evidence base and community knowledge can yield a strong basis for increased use of current evidence-based practices in resource-poor communities.
CPIC: outsider concerns	Partner with trusted community member	Larger community may view community member as selling out	Conduct partnered meetings and trainings at community sites to obtain community feedback throughout project
Recognition of input	Include community and academic members as co-authors and celebrate products	Author order may be a source of tension, especially among academics; community products may be unfamiliar to academics	Dissemination activities such as co-authored presentations and papers enhance the likelihood of reaching critical audiences and lend validity to future efforts and thus future products, while building trust and respect in the partnership
MHIT/PRC: disseminating findings	Publication of a special issue	Delays in finalizing manuscripts due to large partnerships as authors	Designate a single point-person to field questions, circulate drafts of manuscripts and integrate partner feedback

roots" or unaffiliated community members. For W4W, the open meetings in the community attracted many unaffiliated community members into early leadership roles.

For MHIT, the urgency and commonality of the disaster experience mobilized many providers as well as informal community leaders such as those from faith-based organizations. For CPIC, because it was conducted as a partnered research initiative with broad reach into diverse community-based organizations, community members and staff of diverse organizations stepped into leadership and group member roles early on. LACCDR as directed from a policy/services agency has somewhat greater representation of agency leaders and responders. A lesson learned here is that the public health department had to undergo an internal culture change to fully embrace and align with a community partnered approach to building resilience. Across all projects, many agency leaders and responders served dual roles as persons directly affected by disasters or stressors. Thus across projects, the salience of distinguishing between community leader, member, and even researcher is often blurred. It has been learned that these multiple roles are beneficial in setting project goals and can make them more community relevant by asking individuals for their own goals from multiple perspectives: personal, agency, or community.

Policymakers and funders: for policymakers as well as funders, a key lesson learned is the time required to establish and maintain authentic partnerships, whether for services, research, or both and within those partnerships to tackle substantial, sensitive issues such as concerns with depression or psychological consequences of trauma. Especially in the context of vulnerable populations, the level of trust development required and "insider-outsider" dynamics following disasters, necessitate an approach that is responsive to urgent needs as well as feasible but also takes a long-term view of the value of relationships and investments in mental health. Fortunately, in the projects described by the authors, the support of funding agencies and policymakers to explore how to achieve a community engagement focus within their work and any measure of success that they have achieved are due in no small part to their support. For LACCDR, the fact that public health policymakers committed at the outset to this direction has been quite important as we face the challenges inherent in blending perspectives of responders, community members, traditional providers and community leaders, and evaluators.

Overall, our "tale of 2 cities" has suggested that diverse partnerships can organize around goals to improve community and individual outcomes. The authors have learned the many lessons shared here in applying this model to address mental health problems and disaster recovery and are now in the early stages of applying this model to preparedness and community resiliency.

ACKNOWLEDGMENTS

The authors wish to thank their partners for making this work possible. This work was supported by NIH Research Grant # P30MH082760 and R01MH078853 funded by the National Institute of Mental Health, Red Cross Grant # BHGP-08-006 and CDC Grant # 2U90TP917012-11.

REFERENCES

1. Chandra A, Acosta JD. Disaster recovery also involves human recovery. JAMA 2010;304(14):1608.
2. Hobfoll S, Watson P, Bell C, et al. Five essential elements of immediate and mid-term mass trauma intervention: empirical evidence. Psychiatry 2007;70(4): 283–315.

3. Moore M, Chandra A, Acosta J. Building community resilience: what can the United States learn from experiences in other countries? Disaster Med Public Health Prep, in press.

4. Norris FH, Friedman MJ, Watson PJ, et al. 60,000 disaster victims speak: part I. An empirical review of the empirical literature, 1981–2001. Psychiatry 2002; 65(3):207–39.

5. Reissman DB. New roles for mental and behavioral health experts to enhance emergency preparedness and response readiness. Psychiatry 2004;67(2): 118–22.

6. Kessler R, Galea S, Gruber M, et al. Trends in mental illness and suicidality after Hurricane Katrina. Mol Psychiatry 2008;13(4):374–84.

7. Neria Y, Galea S. Post-traumatic stress disorder following disasters: a systematic review. Psychol Med 2008;38(4):467–80.

8. Institute of Medicine. Preparing for the psychological consequences of terrorism: a public health strategy. Washington, DC: National Academy Press; 2003.

9. King M, Schreiber M, Formanski S, et al. Surveillance of traumatic experiences and exposures after the earthquake-A brief report of tsunami in American Samoa, 2009. Disaster Med Public Health Prep, 2012 [Epub ahead of print].

10. Abramson D, Stehling-Ariza T, Garfield R, et al. Prevalence and predictors of mental health distress post-Katrina: findings from the Gulf Coast Child and Family Health Study. Disaster Med Public Health Prep 2008;2(2):77–86.

11. Benight C, Ironson G, Durham R. Psychometric properties of a hurricane coping self-efficacy measure. J Trauma Stress 1999;12(2):379–86.

12. Joshi P, Lewin S. Disaster, terrorism, and children: addressing the effects of traumatic events on children and their families is critical to long-term recovery and resilience. Psychiatr Ann 2004;34(9):710–6.

13. Acosta J, Chandra A, Feeney KC. Navigating the road to recovery: assessment of the coordination, communication, and financing of the disaster case management pilot in Louisiana. Arlington, VA: Rand Corp; 2010.

14. Chandra A, Acosta J. The role of nongovernmental organizations in long-term human recovery after disaster: reflections from Louisiana four years after Hurricane Katrina, vol. 277. Arlington, VA: Rand Corp; 2009.

15. Sinclair J, Bixler D, Cummings KJ, et al. Displacement of the underserved: medical needs of Hurricane Katrina evacuees in West Virginia. J Health Care Poor Underserved 2007;18(2):369–81.

16. Davis JR, Wilson S, Brock-Martin A, et al. The impact of disasters on populations with health and health care disparities. Disaster Med Public Health Prep 2010; 4(1):30.

17. Hobfoll S, Palmieri P, Johnson R, et al. Trajectories of resilience, resistance, and distress during ongoing terrorism: the case of Jews and Arabs in Israel. J Consult Clin Psychol 2009;77(1):138–48.

18. Schoenbaum M, Butler B, Kataoka S, et al. Promoting mental health recovery after Hurricanes Katrina and Rita: what can be done at what cost. Arch Gen Psychiatry 2009;66(8):906–14.

19. Wang P, Gruber M, Powers R, et al. Mental health service use among Hurricane Katrina survivors in the eight months after the disaster. Psychiatr Serv 2007; 58(11):1403–11.

20. Everly GS Jr, Phillips SB, Kane D, et al. Introduction to and overview of group psychological first aid. Brief Treatment and Crisis Intervention 2006;6(2):130.

21. Federal Emergency Management Agency. National disaster recovery framework: Strengthening disaster recovery for the nation. Washington DC: Department of Homeland Security. FEMA; 2011. p. 1–116.
22. U.S. Dept of Health and Human Services. National health security strategy of the United States of America. Washington, DC: U.S. Dept of Health and Human Services; 2009.
23. Pfefferbaum R, Reissman D, Pfefferbaum B, et al. Factors in the development of community resilience to disasters. Cambridge (United Kingdom): Cambridge University Press; 2008.
24. Kim S, Flaskerud JH, Koniak-Griffin D, et al. Using community-partnered participatory research to address health disparities in a Latino community. J Prof Nurs 2005;21(4):199–209.
25. Nyamathi A, Koniak-Griffin D, Ann Greengold B. Development of nursing theory and science in vulnerable populations research. Annu Rev Nurs Res 2007;25(1): 3–25.
26. Pieters HC, Heilemann MS, Grant M, et al. Older women's reflections on accessing care across their breast cancer trajectory: navigating beyond the triple barriers. Oncol Nurs Forum 2011;38(2):175–84.
27. Pieters HC, Heilemann MS, Maliski S, et al. Instrumental relating and treatment decision making among older women with early stage breast cancer. Oncol Nurs Forum, in Press.
28. Minkler M. Community-based participatory research for health. San Francisco (CA): Jossey-Bass; 2003.
29. Watkins K, Paddock S, Zhang L, et al. Improving care for depression in patients with comorbid substance misuse. American Journal of Psychiatry 2006;163(1):125–32.
30. Institute of Medicine. Promoting health: intervention strategies from social and behavioral research. Washington, DC: National Academy Press; 2000.
31. Israel B, Eng E, Schulz A, et al. Methods in community-based participatory research for health. San Francisco (CA): Jossey-Bass; 2005.
32. Smedley BD, Syme SL. Promoting health: intervention strategies from social and behavioral research. Washington, DC: National Academies Press; 2000.
33. Tunis S, Stryer D, Clancy C. Practical clinical trials: increasing the value of clinical research for decision making in clinical and health policy. JAMA 2003; 290(12):1624–32.
34. Wells K, Miranda J, Bruce M, et al. Bridging community intervention and mental health services research. Am J Psychiatry 2004;161(6):955–63.
35. Zerhouni E. Translational and clinical science–time for a new vision. N Engl J Med 2005;353(15):1621–3.
36. Zerhouni E. US biomedical research: basic, translational, and clinical sciences. JAMA 2005;294(11):1352–8.
37. Jones L, Wells K, Norris K, et al. The vision, valley, and victory of community engagement. Ethn Dis 2009;19(Suppl):S6-3–7.
38. Wells K, Jones L. "Research" in community-partnered, participatory research. JAMA 2009;302(3):320–1.
39. Bluthenthal R, Jones L, Fackler-Lowrie N, et al. Witness for wellness: preliminary findings from a community-academic participatory research mental health initiative. Ethn Dis 2006;16(Suppl):S18–34.
40. Chung B, Jones L, Dixon E, et al. Community Partners in Care Steering Council. Using a community partnered participatory research approach to implement a randomized controlled trial: planning community partners in care. J Health Care Poor Underserved 2010;21(3):780–95.

41. Miranda J, Ong MK, Jones L, et al. Community-partnered evaluation of depression services for clients of community-based agencies in under-resourced communities in Los Angeles. Journal of General Internal Medicine 2013. http://dx.doi.org/10.1007/s11606-013-2480-7.

42. Wells KB, Jones L, Chung B, et al. Community-partnered cluster-randomized comparative effectiveness trial of community engagement and planning or resources for services to address depression disparities. Journal of General Internal Medicine 2013. http://dx.doi.org/10.1007/s11606-013-2484-3.

43. Springgate B, Wennerstrom A, Meyers D, et al. Building community resilience through mental health infrastructure and training in post-Katrina New Orleans. Ethn Dis 2011;21(Suppl 1):S1-20–9.

44. Lizaola E, Schraiber R, Braslow J, et al. The Partnered Research Center for Quality Care: developing infrastructure to support community-partnered participatory research in mental health. Ethn Dis 2011;21(3 Suppl 1):S1.

45. Ford CL, Airhihenbuwa CO. Critical race theory, race equity, and public health: toward antiracism praxis. Am J Public Health 2010;100(Suppl 1):S30–5.

46. Thomas SB, Quinn SC, Butler J, et al. Toward a fourth generation of disparities research to achieve health equity. Annu Rev Public Health 2011;32:399–416.

47. Chung B, Corbett CE, Boulet B, et al. Talking wellness: a description of a community-academic partnered project to engage an African-American community around depression through the use of poetry, film, and photography. Ethn Dis 2006;16(1):S67–78.

48. Patel KK, Koegel P, Booker T, et al. Innovative approaches to obtaining community feedback in the Witness for Wellness experience. Ethn Dis 2006;16(1):S35–42.

49. Stockdale S, Patel K, Gray R, et al. Supporting wellness through policy and advocacy: a case history of a working group in a community partnership initiative to address depression. Ethn Dis 2006;16(1):S43–53.

50. Jones D, Franklin C, Butler BT, et al. The Building Wellness Project: a case history of partnership, power sharing, and compromise. Ethn Dis 2006;16(1):S54–6.

51. Wells KB, Sherbourne C, Schoenbaum M, et al. Impact of disseminating quality improvement programs for depression in managed primary care. JAMA 2000;283(2):212.

52. Chung B, Jones L, Jones A, et al. Using community arts events to enhance collective efficacy and community engagement to address depression in an African American community. Am J Public Health 2009;99(2):237.

53. Jones L, Wells K. Strategies for academic and clinician engagement in community-participatory partnered research. JAMA 2007;297(4):407–10.

54. Voelker R. Robert Wood Johnson Clinical Scholars Mark 35 Years of Health Services Research. JAMA 2007;297(23):2571–3.

55. Miranda J, Chung JY, Green BL, et al. Treating depression in predominantly low-income young minority women. JAMA 2003;290(1):57–65.

56. Unützer J, Katon W, Callahan CM, et al. Collaborative care management of late-life depression in the primary care setting. JAMA 2002;288(22):2836–45.

57. Wennerstrom A, Vannoy SD, Allen C. Community-based participatory development of a community health worker mental health outreach role to extend collaborative care in post-Katrina New Orleans. Ethn Dis 2011;21(Suppl 1):S1–45.

58. Katz DL, Murimi M, Gonzalez A, et al. From controlled trial to community adoption: the multisite translational community trial. Am J Public Health 2011;101(8):e17–27.

59. Wells KB, Tang J, Lizaola E, et al. Applying community engagement to disaster planning: developing the vision and design for the Los Angeles County Community Disaster Resilience initiative. Am J Public Health 2013;103(7):1172–80.

60. Plough A, Fielding JE, Chandra A, et al. Building community disaster resilience: perspectives from a large urban county department of public health. Am J Public Health 2013;103(7):1190–7.

61. Chandra A, Williams M, Plough A, et al. Getting actionable about community resilience: the Los Angeles County Community Disaster Resilience project. Am J Public Health 2013;103(7):1181–9.

62. Woodward A. Long-term oil disaster study still seeks participants. Available at: http://www.bestofneworleans.com/blogofneworleans/archives/2012/10/02/long-term-oil-disaster-study-still-seeks-participants. Accessed December 15, 2012.

Index

Note: Page numbers of article titles are in **boldface** type.

Psychiatr Clin N Am 36 (2013) 467–474
http://dx.doi.org/10.1016/S0193-953X(13)00078-6
0193-953X/13/$ – see front matter © 2013 Elsevier Inc. All rights reserved.

psych.theclinics.com

Moving?

Make sure your subscription moves with you!

To notify us of your new address, find your **Clinics Account Number** (located on your mailing label above your name), and contact customer service at:

Email: journalscustomerservice-usa@elsevier.com

800-654-2452 (subscribers in the U.S. & Canada)
314-447-8871 (subscribers outside of the U.S. & Canada)

Fax number: 314-447-8029

Elsevier Health Sciences Division
Subscription Customer Service
3251 Riverport Lane
Maryland Heights, MO 63043

*To ensure uninterrupted delivery of your subscription, please notify us at least 4 weeks in advance of move.

Printed and bound by CPI Group (UK) Ltd, Croydon, CR0 4YY

03/10/2024

01040409-0016